UNICORN PARTS AND GLITTER

QUICK AND DIRTY TIPS FOR SURVIVING A J-POUCH

A.W. CROSS

GLORY BOX PRESS

Unicorn Farts and Glitter: Quick and Dirty Tips for Surviving a J-Pouch

Cover illustration by Peter Cross
Cover design by germancreative
Book design and production by Glory Box Press
Editing by Mia Darien

A.W. Cross
gloryboxpress@gmail.com

Printed in Canada

First Printing: August 2016

ISBN 978-0-9950991-5-9

ABOUT THE AUTHOR

A.W. Cross is a Canadian writer and blogger and has experienced nearly everything a j-pouch has to offer. Whenever she has time, she enjoys her family, friends, and reliving the glory days of Star Trek and the Golden Girls.

You can follow her on Facebook @thescreamingmeemie or visit her website, screamingmeemie.com

Unicorn Farts and Glitter: Quick and Dirty Tips for Surviving a J-Pouch is her third book.

Other Titles in the *Quick and Dirty Tips for Surviving* Series:

You Don't Look Sick: Quick and Dirty Tips for Surviving Ulcerative Colitis
Unicorn Farts and Glitter: Quick and Dirty Tips for Surviving a J-Pouch

For all j-pouchers: may our farts smell like rainbows and echo like a unicorn's laughter.

CONTENTS

PREFACE

I was diagnosed with ulcerative colitis in 2009. A little over three years later my colon was gone, and I was the owner of a shiny new j-pouch. I was cured. Only, I wasn't. No one tells you how long your recovery will truly take. *Six weeks*, the doctors say. What they *should* tell you is *six weeks, plus another forty-six, give or take*. Six weeks and I could get out of bed, sure, but it wasn't until an entire year had passed that I began to feel as though I was really recovering. And I was a best-case scenario. No complications, no urgency to return to work, no children to chase. I was extremely lucky.

It wasn't until the third year after my surgery that I could say I felt *well*. But even though my recovery was long and painful, it was also wonderful. I had adjusted to my ileostomy, even *liked* it, but with my j-pouch, I felt like I had been given a second chance.

No longer encumbered by an external appliance, I fooled myself into thinking that this was it—I had paid my dues, and now I could just get on with life. Then came a bout of pouchitis. And another. And I realized that, despite outward appearances, I was never going to be "normal" again. And at that point, after everything I had been through, my only options were to laugh or cry.

I did both. But I laughed more.

In 2015 (now sans ostomy), I joined the NaNoWriMo rebellion, and I wrote what would eventually become three books—this is the third. Writing about what I learned during my illness also inspired me to found my IBD blog, screamingmeemie.com.

I hope this book makes you smile and your recovery even a little bit easier. I know it did mine.

A.W. Cross, 2016

INTRODUCTION

Congratulations! You've defeated whatever condition robbed you of your colon, dominated an ostomy, and come out the other side. You have been rebuilt. They had the technology. They made you better than you were. Stronger, faster. Or at the very least, able to fart again.

You are now among the elite. Seasoned, adaptable, and able to employ unconventional skills and methods to ensure your survival. You are a figure of medical legend, blending in seamlessly with society as you continue your battle against an invisible foe. You may be forgiven for thinking that you have paid your dues, that now is your time to rest. It is not.

Your primary goal is to achieve confidence, continence, and healthy perianal skin. This book will help you achieve these objectives by instructing you on the use of bulking agents, proper skin care, and the art of dryly passing gas. You will be prepared to recognize the signs of pouchitis and obstructions and learn how to respond swiftly and effectively. You will be schooled in talking about your illness on social media, how to adapt in a hospital situation, and how to deal with hostile non-pouchers.

Although this book will touch on medical aspects of your j-pouch, that is not its focus. Instead, the aim is to equip you with the means to cope with the mental and physical consequences of having a j-pouch, from post-traumatic stress to why you should never wear polyester underwear.

Navigating the unpredictable landscape of your new body is not easy, and this book won't change that. Use it as a starting point, drawing on knowledge hard-won from years of personal experience.

Welcome, comrade, to the other side.

J-POUCH

UNICORN FARTS AND GLITTER

LIABILITIES OF A J-POUCH

Before you get all cocky with your newly-gotten pooping-through-your-bum-again fabulousness, having an internal pouch has its own set of drawbacks:

BUTT BURN

You'll become well-acquainted with the feeling of firing sizzling-hot artillery out of your ass. This anal scorching is due to both the digestive enzymes in your stool (the very same ones that burned your peristomal skin when you had an ostomy) and the phenomenon that food comes out spicier than it went in.

BLOCKAGES

You'll continue to have issues with intestinal obstructions—blockages from adhesions are even more likely due to your increased scar tissue.

POUCHITIS

Your pouch will occasionally become inflamed, requiring a course of antibiotics. If you have persistent pouchitis, you may need to have more intensive treatment or have your pouch reversed back into an ileostomy.

SCARS

You will have a large, vertical abdominal scar and a smaller, horizontal ostomy scar.

DIARRHEA
Welcome back, old friend. Some days you will go to the toilet four times a day, some days it will be fourteen. Almost like bowel disease. Again. Yay.

FATIGUE
Your days will now seem to have thirty-six looooong hours in them.

SKIN DEGRADATION
Your perianal skin (the skin around your no-no) will get damaged even more quickly than your peristomal skin since it's more difficult to prevent your waste from touching it.

HEALTHCARE IGNORANCE
Few general practitioners know how to deal with pouch issues. In general medicine, j-pouchers are like unicorns. Your doctor may prescribe you an obligatory course of antibiotics whether you have pouchitis or not, or they may refuse to treat you and will simply refer you to a specialist.

REDUCED FERTILITY
Due to scar tissue webbing on your fallopian tubes, conceiving can be more difficult. If you don't want to get pregnant, congratulations— free birth control. (Warning: very unpredictable.)

DEHYDRATION
Since you absorb most water and salts with your colon, and a j-pouch is not (despite all intents and purposes) a colon, you'll continue to get dehydrated easily.

LONG RECOVERY AND ADJUSTMENT PERIOD
Think of your recovery in terms of months and years, rather than weeks.

ASSETS OF A J-POUCH

Now for the good stuff:

YOU CAN FART AGAIN

With caution. Please refer to Chapter Three.

BRAND-NEW BUTTHOLE

Even if nobody ever sees it (yourself included), enjoy the knowledge that you got a spanking-new, sparkling-fresh, maximum-sphincter butthole. For free. People pay to have that stuff done, and you got it FOR FREE.

SCARS

Badass, hero-survivor scars.

MEDICATION

Or lack thereof. Definitely less than when you had active disease.

NO MORE STOMA

Having a stoma is a Good Thing, but it can require a lot of upkeep. You'll miss it, even if just for its ability to let you eat as much spicy food as you want. You'll *especially* miss it when you have pouchitis.

SOCIAL CURRENCY

When people find out about your internal pouch, they think you're proper hard-core. Or a freak of medical science. There is no need to disabuse them of either notion—be mysterious.

BATTLE SCARS

PHYSICAL CONSEQUENCES OF A J-POUCH

PHYSICAL CONSEQUENCES OF A J-POUCH AND HOW TO COPE

The important thing for you to remember about recovering from your internal pouch surgery is that your recovery is a marathon, not a sprint. You are recovering not only from major surgery—or more likely, multiple surgeries within a short period—but your pouch itself takes a long time to adapt. You shouldn't consider your physical recovery in terms of weeks or even months, but *years*. This does not mean years of complications, but it does take a minimum of a year, even in the best case scenario, until your pouch adjusts and you begin to feel "normal."

Many of the physical issues associated with having an internal pouch you'll already be familiar with, but some may be new:

SCARRING
You will have greater internal and external scarring.

FATIGUE
You will find yourself getting tired easily.

SKIN IRRITATION AND DEGRADATION
You will be surprised at how quickly and easily your perianal skin can become compromised.

VITAMIN AND MINERAL DEFICIENCY

Malabsorption and your potential inability to eat certain foods can cause you to become deficient in elements such as potassium.

LOOSE STOOL

Your stool will be liquid on a bad day, semi-formed the rest of the time. You may find you are moderately incontinent at first and experience minor leakage.

FREQUENT STOOL

Initially, you will probably go to the toilet ten to twenty times per day. After six months, this frequency should reduce to five to ten times per day, and after one to two years, you will likely be going only three to five times per day. Frequency, of course, will vary between individuals, and you might be the lucky bastard who ends up going only once per day.

In the early days, you may also find you need to go several times during the night, but this too should reduce over time. Your pouch will eventually expand, and its carrying capacity will increase.

ABDOMINAL CRAMPING

If you delay going to the bathroom, you may get a brief wave of cramping in your abdomen and rectum.

POSITIONAL PAIN

You may find that lying on one side or the other, or on your stomach, is painful and prompts a strong need to empty your pouch.

WEAKER ABDOMINAL MUSCLES

You've had a lot of surgery there. Give yourself ample time to build your muscles back up, and don't be surprised if they're never quite the same.

BOISTEROUS BOWEL MOVEMENTS

Loud. Explosive. But mercifully brief.

DEHYDRATION
You will become dehydrated quickly.

WEIGHT FLUCTUATIONS
You may find that your appetite is erratic as you recover.

POTENTIAL COMPLICATIONS

There are a number of potential complications associated with having a j-pouch. Although each of the following problems may not become serious, they all warrant a degree of medical care. Consult your physician if you experience any of the following:

OBSTRUCTION
Your bowel will become blocked and unable to pass waste. Blockages are caused by food particles, scar tissue adhesions, and strictures.

POUCHITIS
Pouchitis occurs when your pouch becomes inflamed. Your symptoms will be similar to inflammatory bowel disease, including cramping and diarrhea. Pouchitis is treated with antibiotics.

ADHESIONS
Adhesions occur when the scar tissue caused by your surgeries creates a webbing around and between your organs, causing abdominal pain when they pull or get caught. Obstructions can occur if the adhesions form a stricture (narrowing of your intestine). Severe adhesions must be surgically removed.

SEXUAL DYSFUNCTION
Sexual dysfunction (temporary and permanent) can occur in both men and women, causing symptoms such as reduced libido, erectile dysfunction, vaginal dryness, and pain during intercourse.

REDUCED FERTILITY

You may find your ability to conceive is significantly reduced, resulting in the need for medical intervention. Or, in some cases, infertility.

INCONTINENCE

Although usually temporary, you may find you have a small degree of permanent incontinence.

LEAK AT ANAL CONNECTION

A leak at the connection of your pouch and anus can result in a pelvic abscess or an infection in your abdomen. Both are serious conditions and require medical attention.

ONGOING FREQUENT BOWEL MOVEMENTS

Your bowel frequency should slow as you heal. However, you may find you still need to go frequently.

FISTULAS

Fistulas occur due to inflammation and result in channels between your j-pouch and other organs, such as your vagina.

FISSURES

You'll literally get cracks in your crack. Painful, itchy, and annoying, but not serious unless they become infected.

CUFFITIS

If even a shred of your original rectal tissue is left behind after your colectomy, it can become inflamed. With ulcerative colitis. Again.

DE NOVO CROHN'S DISEASE OF THE POUCH

A small percentage of people develop Crohn's disease in their pouch. Symptoms include weight loss, abdominal pain, nausea, anemia, and fistulas.

POUCH FAILURE

Sometimes, your pouch will simply fail to thrive. You may find it doesn't retain stool, or you have difficulty emptying it when it's full. Pouch failure results in a permanent ostomy.

TIPS FOR COPING

KNOW THE SYMPTOMS OF POUCHITIS
And treat it as soon as you can. Ask your doctor to give you an anticipatory prescription, prescribe refills that you can order directly from the pharmacy as needed, or prescribe enough excess pills for a two or three day supply so you can begin treatment while waiting to see them.

KNOW WHEN TO SEEK HELP
Know the symptoms of serious complications and don't delay seeking help.

CONFIRM ABSORPTION
Ensure your vitamins and any other medications will be absorbed before they exit your pouch by avoiding sustained-release formulas, crushing or breaking your tablets (check with your pharmacist first), or taking liquid, gel, or gummy formulations. Remind your doctor of absorbency issues when they are prescribing your medication.

If you are unsure whether or not a pill will absorb, put it in a glass of warm water for thiry minutes and see if it dissolves. If it does, you're golden.

BE VIGILANT ABOUT YOUR SKIN CARE
Perianal skin is as delicate as tissue paper, and once it's inflamed, it takes a long time to heal. Liberally using a diaper-rash cream or Vaseline® *after every time you go* can make all the difference.

EAT A BALANCED DIET
Start with reliable, low-risk foods and gradually introduce caution foods to determine how well your pouch will cope.

CHEW EVERYTHING WELL
Avoid getting a blockage through this schoolboy (or girl) error.

ADHERE TO THE FARTING GUIDELINES
Keep your underwear clean and dry, and your face free from blushes.

STAY HYDRATED
Drink lots of fluid and avoid too much direct sunlight. Although it can be tempting to drink little and often, you can train your bowel to absorb greater quantities of fluid over time by drinking larger amounts.

TAKE IT EASY
Avoid strenuous physical activity for at least 12 weeks, then build yourself back up. It's hard to get motivated after everything you've been through, but keep moving forward. Avoid lifting anything remotely heavy for the first three months.

BE GENTLE
Avoid putting pressure on your abdomen. This is especially important for the first few months, but you may find that even years later, any significant amount of pressure can be uncomfortable and painful.

KEEP A JOURNAL
A journal can be helpful to keep track of your progress, especially if you're having issues, by making it easier to spot patterns in your good and bad days.

BE PROACTIVE ABOUT LEAKAGE
If you're having leakage, wear a pad to absorb it. If you're having significant leakage, you may have to go back to diapers until you can get it under control.

DAB, DON'T WIPE
The importance of dabbing cannot be emphasized enough, especially in the beginning.

USE A BULKING AGENT
Psyllium (such as Metamucil®), methylcellulose (Citrucel®), and calcium polycarbophil (FiberCon®) can add bulk to your stool.

TAKE AN ANTIDIARRHEAL
Medications such as Imodium® can be useful to help slow down your movements. Take only as directed, and check with your doctor if you plan to use them on a long-term, regular basis. Avoid Imodium® when you have pouchitis.

EAT SMALL AMOUNTS OF FOOD, OFTEN
You'll find it easier to digest smaller amounts, which can minimize bloating, improve your nutrition, and help prevent blockages.

HOLD IT
The urgency you feel to go to the bathroom will diminish over time as your pouch expands. Practice holding it for increasingly longer periods (minutes at first, not hours). Holding it in can also help make your stool bulkier and "drier."

RELEARN HOW TO USE THE TOILET
You may have to sit on the toilet for a good few minutes for your pouch to empty properly. This will also improve over time. If you feel your pouch is not emptying completely, you can bear down if you need to, but GENTLY. Sometimes just standing up will help shift things, as does rocking on the toilet seat. Take advantage of any positional pressure if you need to, but only as a last resort.

NEVER USE LAXATIVES
Drink coffee instead.

BE PATIENT
Pouch function, strength, sexuality, appetite—all take time to improve.

CAN'T WAIT: ACCESS TO PUBLIC BATHROOMS

Although knowledge about j-pouches is increasing, the public services that support them vary between countries.

Through Crohn's and Colitis UK, j-pouchers are eligible for a *Can't Wait Card*, a wallet-size card which indicates the holder has a medical condition resulting in an urgency to use the bathroom. The cards encourage businesses to grant the holder access to washrooms that may not be available to the general public. Also available for UK patients is the *RADAR* key. Produced by the National Key Scheme, the key can be used to unlock public bathrooms all over the UK.

Crohn's and Colitis Australia also supports a *Can't Wait* program, which supplies cards to patient members, and *Can't Wait* stickers to businesses and retailers who display the stickers in their windows, indicating to cardholders that their toilets are available when needed. *Can't Wait Cards* are also available in the United States through the Crohn's and Colitis Foundation of America.

At the time of writing, Canada's *Can't Wait* program is still in its infancy. Services currently available include the *GoHere Washroom Finder App*, which uses GPS to locate a washroom nearby and which can also be used to map out locations along a route of travel. There currently is no physical *Can't Wait Card* in Canada, but a virtual *GoHere Washroom Access Card* is available via the *Washroom Finder* app. A *GoHere* decal, similar to Australia's *Can't Wait* sticker, is also on trial in several Canadian cities, with plans to go nationwide if the pilot is successful.

THE WINDS OF CHANGE

THE ART OF FARTING (AND NOT SHARTING)

Although it's extremely exciting to finally be able to fart again, successfully breaking wind is an art that must be learned and practiced with caution. As when you had a colon, you will release two kinds of farts, the long and thin, and the short and explosive. Inconveniently, both can result in follow-through known as the shart. Although you do have a sphincter, your farts are no longer surrounded by the pillowy colon which allowed them to pass in a controlled explosion. You will eventually master the technique in the years after your recovery, but while you're a novice, follow these tips:

- Attempt to fart when you are alone—j-pouch farts can be alarmingly funky.
- The first few times you (intentionally) fart, make sure you're sitting on the toilet. It may have been a long time, and your sphincter might be taken by surprise.
- Once you have gained more control over your bowels and anticipate an off-the-toilet attempt, place a protective layer—such as a panty-liner—in your underwear as a security measure.
- Practice farting while lying on your back. Lying down will help keep everything as closed as possible while still letting the fart escape. When you have mastered that, practice on your side. Only then should you attempt to fart while standing.

- For the first standing fart, strategically place some toilet paper or a pantyliner, clench your cheeks together (butt-cheeks, obviously), and let it creep or squeak through.
- Relax your cheeks in increments over the next few episodes.
- You may think that the long and thins will be safer. This is deceptive.
- Even if you have accomplished a dry fart on several occasions, don't get cocky. Cockiness causes reckless sphincters.
- Be especially vigilant about night-farts as they tend to be the most insidious.
- Always keep your legs and/or butt-cheeks together as a safety net.
- If you do follow through, don't let it damage your confidence. It happens to the best of us, and usually more than once.

THE NOSTALGIC ACHE

POUCHITIS, CUFFITIS, OBSTRUCTIONS, STRICTURES, AND SKIN CARE

POUCHITIS

Pouchitis is an inflammation of your j-pouch. If you've had ulcerative colitis, and you're a sucker for nostalgia, you'll enjoy pouchitis—it feels almost like a flare. Statistics on pouchitis vary, but it's safe to say that approximately 25-50% of people with j-pouches will have at least one bout of pouchitis. If you haven't had it yet, don't feel left out—your chances of getting pouchitis increase every year. A bout of pouchitis can be short and sweet, lasting only a couple of weeks, or it can become a chronic condition.

SYMPTOMS OF POUCHITIS

Symptoms of pouchitis may be mild or severe and can include:

- abdominal pain and cramping
- increased frequency of bowel movements
- diarrhea
- tenesmus (constantly feeling like you need to go to the bathroom)
- bloody stool
- nausea and headache (usually due to dehydration)

- incontinence and leakage
- joint pain
- feeling generally unwell

DIAGNOSIS OF POUCHITIS

Your first bout of pouchitis will likely be confirmed by an endoscopy and bloodwork, which will be ordered based on your symptoms. (What? You thought you were done with all that? Ha!) Once you have an official diagnosis for that initial bout, subsequent bouts may be diagnosed by symptoms alone and treated at your doctor's discretion.

TREATMENT OF POUCHITIS

Pouchitis is treated with antibiotics. Most commonly prescribed is a combination therapy of Ciprofloxacin® and Metronizadole®, which are usually effective at relieving symptoms within three days. A normal course of treatment is two weeks, but you may be given a longer course if your symptoms persist. Alternatives to Ciprofloxacin® and Metronizadole® include Rifaximin® and Tinidazole®, and you may be prescribed varying combinations of the four. If your pouchitis becomes particularly severe, you may also be treated with oral, enema, or suppository doses of mesalamine.

If you end up being one of the unlucky few whose pouchitis becomes antibiotic-resistant (refractory), and you have no relief with mesalamine or similar 5-ASAs, then corticosteroid treatments, such as budesonide enemas, may also be considered, as may biologics such as infliximab, or more rarely, procedures such as leukocytopharesis. These methods are not always successful, however, and at some point, you may have to consider returning to an ostomy to maintain a good quality of life.

PREVENTING POUCHITIS

Pouchitis is notoriously difficult to prevent, and there is not, at present, a definitive method that works for everyone. There are numerous theories and suggestions regarding diet, stress, probiotics (such as VSL#3), and various holistic treatments, but these therapies seem to have inconsistent success. The likely reason is that there are multiple factors involved in creating the perfect storm for each bout of pouchitis to occur, and these combinations of factors are unique to the individual at that point in time. Do your research and try whatever methods speak to you. With any luck, one of them will work.

CUFFITIS

Cuffitis is the poor cousin of pouchitis. Also known as rectal cuff inflammation, cuffitis occurs in rectal tissue left behind after your colectomy, even if your surgeon swears he got it all. It is most likely to occur if you had ulcerative colitis and is basically a continuation of the disease. It's uncomfortable and annoying, and, if it's your birthday, it can occur at the same time as pouchitis.

SYMPTOMS OF CUFFITIS

Symptoms of cuffitis include:

- rectal (and sometimes abdominal)pain and pressure
- rectal itching
- increased urgency to go to the bathroom
- bloody bowel movements

DIAGNOSIS OF CUFFITIS

Unfortunately, cuffitis is diagnosed (at least the first time) with either an endoscope, or, if your doctor knows what they're feeling for, a finger. You may be tempted to pass your symptoms off as pouchitis to avoid being probed, but because cuffitis it treated differently than pouchitis, a differential diagnosis is important.

TREATMENT OF CUFFITIS

While treatment for pouchitis relies on the use of antibiotics, cuffitis is typically treated with either mesalamine (such as Pentasa®, Asacol®, or Canasa®) or corticosteroid suppositories and foam enemas.

OBSTRUCTIONS

Obstructions are a serious and extremely painful concern for j-pouchers. Often an obstruction will be only a partial blockage that resolves itself without medical intervention. Other times, obstructions can be more serious and require hospitalization and possibly surgery.

CAUSES OF OBSTRUCTION

Blockages can be caused by:

- Strictures of your intestine due to scar tissue. Strictures commonly occur at the anastomosis site (where your pouch attaches to your anus).
- Adhesions of scar tissue. Scar tissue can adhere your intestine to itself, to your other organs, or to your abdominal wall.
- Kinks or twists in your intestine.
- High-fiber foods (or foods that are otherwise difficult to digest), not chewing your food properly, overeating, and dehydration can all inhibit proper digestion of food and result in an obstruction.

SYMPTOMS OF AN OBSTRUCTION

You may have an obstruction if you:

- feel sharp, gas-like pains (although it may just be gas)
- pass little or no stool for several hours
- feel bloated and full
- experience waves of painful abdominal cramping (if the blockage has not resolved)
- have nausea and vomiting

COPING WITH AN OBSTRUCTION

To try and resolve a blockage yourself:

- Stop eating solids.
- Drink water, coffee, tea, soda, or sports drinks. Fluids may help resolve the blockage, especially if it's due to dehydration.
- DO NOT USE LAXATIVES.
- Sit on the toilet and GENTLY bear down. Do not persist if you have no results in the first minute. Stand up, walk around, then try again. DO NOT strain.
- Rub your belly, and rock either on your hands and knees or your back while holding your knees. These movements can help free a partial blockage and can also shift gas.
- Take a hot bath; it may get things moving again. You can also try a heating pad on your belly.
- If your symptoms continue and you pass no stool for four to six hours, the pain becomes severe, or you begin to vomit, then **go to the hospital.**

PREVENTING AN OBSTRUCTION

You may be able to avoid a blockage if you:

- Avoid foods that you have previously found difficult to digest.
- Eat only small amounts of high-risk foods, and chew them well.
- Chew ALL food well, even if it's not a caution food.

You cannot prevent an obstruction due to strictures and/or adhesions. Knowing the signs and how to cope is the best you can do.

POUCH STRICTURE

Ileal pouch stricture is a specific type of obstruction which causes a narrowing of your pouch either at the outlet (the anastomosis at the bottom end of your pouch), the inlet (the top entrance of your pouch), or of the body of your pouch itself. Some strictures can be resolved with medication or simple dilation, while others require surgery.

CAUSES OF STRICTURES

Pouch stricture can be caused by:

- ischemia (impaired blood flow to the area)
- scar tissue
- inflammation due to conditions such as pouchitis, cuffitis, cuff abscess, or Crohn's disease
- persistent leaks at the anastomosis
- the use of NSAIDS (nonsteroidal anti-inflammatory drugs), which can cause irritation

SYMPTOMS OF STRICTURES

Symptoms of pouch stricture include:

- difficulty passing waste
- cramping and abdominal pain
- bloating
- nausea and vomiting
- diarrhea
- tenesmus

DIAGNOSIS OF STRICTURES

In combination with your symptoms, your doctor will diagnose a pouch stricture either manually (yes, that means with a finger), with an endoscope, or with a barium X-ray.

TREATMENT OF STRICTURES

Treatment of strictures varies according to the cause and location, but may include the following methods:

MEDICATION
If your stricture is caused by inflammation, you will be prescribed anti-inflammatories and antibiotics to resolve the inflammation and reduce the stricture.

MANUAL DILATION
If your stricture is at the outlet (rectal end), your doctor may stretch your anastomosis with their finger(s) or a dilator. You may also be given instructions on how to self-dilate at home. DO NOT ATTEMPT SELF-DILATION WITHOUT PROPER INSTRUCTION OR EQUIPMENT. Seriously, don't. Unless you want to be the subject of the next ER cocktail party.

BALLOON DILATION
A small balloon is inserted endoscopically into the strictured area and inflated gradually over multiple sessions. The procedure is usually performed on those strictures located at either the pouch inlet or the pouch itself. Anesthesia optional but recommended!

SURGERY
If your stricture cannot be resolved by manual or balloon dilation, you may need to have a strictureplasty to remove the scar tissue, or less commonly, your pouch may be resectioned and a new anastomosis formed.

REVERSAL OF J-POUCH
If all the above methods fail to resolve your stricture, you will have to revert to a permanent ostomy.

TIPS FOR COPING WITH A STRICTURE

If you suspect you have a stricture:

- Stop taking bulking agents.
- See your doctor as soon as you can. Waste buildup can cause complications with impaction and infection that can become very serious.
- Do not attempt manual dilation unless you have the proper equipment and have been instructed how to do so safely.
- Do not strain if you cannot pass waste. Straining can cause both ischemia and pouch prolapse.

SKIN CARE

Skin care is paramount when you have a j-pouch. In the first few months to a year, you'll be going to the toilet frequently, and each time your fragile butt-skin is exposed to a litany of excretionary insults. Like your peristomal skin, your perianal skin is easy to damage and hard to repair—you may find yourself living with perpetual diaper rash, despite your best efforts at prevention.

CAUSES OF PERIANAL SKIN DAMAGE

- Your stool is caustic—it's full of digestive enzymes that will happily eat away your skin.
- The aggressiveness of those digestive enzymes is compounded by the frequency with which you pass them.
- Wiping, wiping, wiping. Even if you use the softest toilet paper available, repeated wiping will eventually cause irritation.
- Over-hydration of your skin, especially if you are passing a lot of liquid. Excess moisture makes your skin more fragile and prone to tearing.
- The odd crafty scratch. You think one swipe won't hurt, but your skin can become so delicate that even a light scratch on the outside of your clothes can peel off layers.

TREATMENT OF SKIN DAMAGE

- If your skin has broken down drastically, and you're passing a lot of liquid stool, you may find it necessary to go to the bathroom in the shower. You'll know when you've gotten to that point, and there's no shame in it. It's no different than when you showered with your ostomy uncovered. Cleaning a shower takes a lot less time than your skin does to heal. Hygiene aside, you don't want to add more moisture to your damaged skin than necessary, but as a short-term solution, it provides temporary relief and gives your skin the respite it needs to heal.

- Use good quality, soft toilet paper or alcohol-and-fragrance-free baby wipes.
- A soft cloth and warm water can also work wonders. Just don't use your facecloth.
- If your skin is quite irritated, dab, don't wipe.
- If you have a bidet, then you're golden. Use in lieu of wiping.
- Keep your skin as dry as possible. For ladies, having your period can subsequently be a bit of a nightmare.
- Use a bulking agent to reduce the frequency of your bowel movements and add form to your stool. Adding bulk will also help absorb some of those enzymes.
- If your skin can tolerate a soap or cleanser, choose one that is pH-balanced and as free of chemicals as possible. Look for ones that don't contain synthetic perfume, alcohol, SLS (sodium lauryl sulphate), or lanolin, since these ingredients can act as irritants to broken skin.
- Create a skin barrier with Vaseline® (or other petroleum-based lotion), barrier cream, diaper cream (zinc-based, which protects without adding moisture), or even the skin barrier wipes you used for your peristomal skin. After using the toilet, make sure your skin is clean and dry before you apply the barrier. Reapply as necessary.
- If your skin is very itchy, add baking soda to your bath or apply a mentholated barrier cream such as Calmoseptine® or Gold Bond®.
- If your skin is in rough shape, clean down to skin level (take off the barrier cream completely), only once per day until your skin has begun to repair. Reapply cream as necessary.
- You can also apply peristomal barrier powders to your damaged skin. Dry, powder, then apply a barrier wipe or cream.
- Warmth and moisture on your damaged skin may cause a fungal rash; it will appear as itchy, white pustules. If you do

have a fungal infection, ask your doctor to prescribe an anti-fungal cream.

- If you have minor leakage, absorb with a strategically placed cotton ball. If your leaks are more than a ball's worth, wear a pantyliner to absorb, and ensure you change it often.
- Protect your skin with a barrier cream even when it's healthy, if only with just a swipe of Vaseline.

STAYIN' ALIVE

PLAN AHEAD

J-POUCH SURVIVAL KIT

One of the best ways to cope successfully with your j-pouch is to prepare for eventualities and carry some essentials with you when you're not at home. In the first few months after your surgery, you may be especially prone to frequent bowel movements and minor leaks.

WIPES

If you thought that extra-soft/triple-ply/has-sewn-in-velvet-pillows toilet paper got rough fast when you were ill, it gets rougher even quicker when you have a j-pouch. Your perianal skin can become so tender, it will feel like you're wiping your butt with a backward porcupine. Choose baby wipes that are fragrance and alcohol-free, ideally those made for sensitive skin. Dab, don't wipe, and make sure you dry yourself. Ever see how well wet tissue paper holds together?

VASELINE®

Use Vaseline®, or any other hypoallergenic petroleum-based lotion, as a barrier to protect your skin from all those digestive enzymes. Diaper rash cream (anything zinc-based) also works well. **Remember:** buy two tubs if you're also using it on your lips.

MENTHOLATED CREAM

Mentholated creams such as Calmoseptine® or Gold Bond® are another type of lotion you can use as a barrier cream—the cooling sensation will stop you from craftily rubbing your butt against the couch when you're itchy. If your cream is very thick, mix it with a looser cream to avoid dragging on your skin when you apply it. Make sure you check the label if you are sensitive to lanolin. Mix with Vaseline® for added protection.

ANTIDIARRHEALS
Such as Imodium®, for emergencies.

PAINKILLERS
Maybe not necessary, but still good to have on hand. Avoid ibuprofen.

A CHANGE OF UNDERWEAR
Unless you're having a bout of full-blown pouchitis, you shouldn't have any leakage so serious it requires a change of pants. Probably.

JUST CHANGE
You may end up being somewhere civilization has forgot, and that has only pay toilets.

SCENT SPRAY
To be honest, your smell is not going to be any worse than anyone else's, just more frequent. If you are feeling self-conscious, however, buy an odor-neutralizing spray, such as anything Poo-pourri™, rather than a cover-up scent. There are also products such as YouGoGirl™, a powder that you sprinkle on top of the water before you go. The powder turns in to foam, and not only does it provide a nice, fresh scent, it also muffles the sound *and* cleans the bowl.

PANTYLINERS
Liners are very useful if you're having a bit of leakage. If you tend to have a lot of leakage, opt for incontinence pads or adult diapers instead.

ANTIBACTERIAL HAND WIPES/GEL
You never know if there will be soap. There might not even be a

bathroom. If you suddenly get extremely itchy, you can swipe yourself with some cooling cream and still be reasonably hygienic until you can get to a sink.

MOISTURIZER
You may be washing your hands a lot.

BULKING SACHETS OR TABLETS
Hauling around a giant can of Metamucil® is not realistic, so if you're going to be out all day, sachets or tablets are a better option. Or, put some in a tiny Tupperware® container, just don't try to take it through airport security.

A LIST OF YOUR CONDITION, MEDICATION, AND DOCTOR'S DETAILS
Just in case you are rendered unconscious, fall down a well, or otherwise need to communicate your extensive needs.

SURVIVAL KIT TIPS

- Have several kits if you can. Keep one at work, one in the car, and one at your local pub. That way, you never have to worry about forgetting it.
- Keep everything together in a separate, dedicated bag. (Don't just fill up your purse or man-bag with items.)
- Keep your kit in an easily accessible location.
- If you don't want to carry full sizes of products or buy travel-sized items, the dollar store is a great place to get various sizes of small bottles and containers.
- Keep anything that might spill or open in separate baggies within your kit.

ADULT DIAPERS: NOT JUST A FETISH

Adult diapers get a lot of flack. Seen as the purview of the very young and the elderly, many teenagers and adults feel uncomfortable and even ashamed at the thought of having to wear a diaper during a bout of pouchitis. It's true that you can navigate these episodes without ever stepping into one. But honestly? Diapers can make your life a hell of a lot easier. I never thought of myself as someone who would ever wear diapers; I saw it as the surrender of the last tattered shred of my feminine dignity.

One day, I had the choice of either missing a special social occasion and staying home next to the toilet, or putting on a diaper and going boldly. After much deliberation, I chose the latter. It was a revelation. I went out for the first time in ages and *enjoyed* myself because I didn't have to worry about having an accident. Don't get me wrong. I did, several times—this was only two weeks after my j-pouch construction—but nobody noticed. Not a single person guessed that I was not only wearing a diaper, but had made good use of it. It actually seemed like people were much more concerned with what they were doing than what I may or may not have had on under my clothes. Funny that.

I only wish that I had gotten over the self-imposed stigma of wearing a diaper sooner. I feel no small regret when I think of all the things I missed doing when I had active ulcerative colitis and chose to stay home rather than wear something that no one else could see. And really, soiling the diaper wasn't a big deal. You make a mess; you clean it up, and you move on. Incontinence can be a fact of life when you have this condition, and there's no shame in it.

Besides, diapers are not for just the very young, old, infirm, or sexually experimental. They are also a staple of occupational wear. Want to know who else wears diapers?

- actors
- professional gamers
- surgeons and nurses
- astronauts

- scuba divers
- pilots
- political figures (during filibustering, for example)
- competitive weightlifters
- guards
- military personnel
- brides (yes, your wedding day is technically the first day of a new job)

So, you're in good company. If a diaper is good enough for a bride to wear on her wedding day, it's good enough for you.

—

I'VE GOT A LOVELY BUNCH OF COCONUTS

WHAT TO PUT IN YOUR MOUTH

J-POUCH DIET DOS AND DON'TS

When it comes to eating, concerns about your j-pouch revolve around avoiding an obstruction and trying to keep your perianal skin intact by regulating what comes out and how often. The following list is not an exact science. You may find every day is different, especially in the beginning. One day you may be able to eat jalapeno popcorn, the next day, even a banana will make you cry.

J-POUCH DIET DOS

- Enjoy foods on the "Don'ts" list, just enjoy them with caution.
- Enjoy everything not on the "Don'ts" list.
- Keep a food diary. An account of what you eat and how you feel over the course of a few months can help you to figure out which foods are compatible with your pouch. You may find that acceptable foods vary from what you could and couldn't tolerate with your ostomy.
- Eat slowly and chew your food well.
- Drink lots of fluids; you'll still be prone to dehydration.

- Eat fruit and vegetables. You may find you can't eat large amounts, especially if they are raw. If they are particularly fibrous, peel and/or cook them lightly first.
- Eat a low-residue diet for the first few weeks until your pouch has adjusted.
- Re-introduce higher-fiber foods one at a time and in small amounts.
- Try a dose of bulking agent thirty minutes before you eat, such as Metamucil® or other similar fiber drink.
- If you need structure, try different diet plans. For example, some j-pouchers have reported success with the FODMAP diet. Just make sure you do your research first.

TIPS

IF YOU'RE CONSTIPATED
Increase your intake of coffee, fruit juice, water, fruit, and vegetables. Increase gradually—you want to get things moving again, but not too much.

IF YOU HAVE DIARRHEA
Try slowing things down with bulking agents, applesauce, bananas, peanut butter, boiled white rice, mashed potato, tapioca, toasted bread, or marshmallows.

J-POUCH DIET DON'TS (OR RATHER, DO, BUT WITH CAUTION)

Slowly introduce these foods back into your diet until you know how your pouch will cope with them. Some of these foods are fibrous and thus difficult to digest. Others cause gas, diarrhea, or the dreaded 'ring of fire.'

FOODS THAT CAN CAUSE OBSTRUCTION

- dried fruit, fruit peels, and fruits such as pineapple, coconut, and oranges
- high-fiber and starchy vegetables such as mushrooms, celery, whole corn, raw cabbage, bean sprouts, and water chestnuts
- nuts, popcorn, and seeds

FOODS THAT CAUSE GAS

- vegetables including cabbage, beans, onions, radishes, cauliflower, cucumber, and soy
- milk
- alcohol, especially beer
- carbonated beverages
- nuts
- chewing gum

Bonus Tip: Drinking through a straw introduces air into your gut that then has to find a way out.

FOODS THAT MAY CAUSE DIARRHEA

- most raw vegetables, leafy greens, cooked cabbage (let's agree just to avoid cabbage)
- most raw fruits, prunes, and raisins
- alcohol
- fried and fatty foods
- whole grains
- bran cereal
- milk
- crab and lobster
- spices

FOODS THAT CAUSE BUTT-BURN AND ARE OTHERWISE ANALLY IRRITATING

- spicy foods
- nuts
- seeds

TIP

DON'T try to be clever or daring with foods that can cause obstructions. Nothing tastes as good as an unblocked intestine feels. Exercise caution when reintroducing these foods, and avoid if you find you have trouble with them. Some people can eat all the coconut they want and drink beer like a sailor, while others can merely look at a beansprout and end up in the hospital. Just make sure you start with small amounts and chew everything well.

IT'S BEETS!

Given your frequent brushes with intestinal and rectal bleeding, you can be forgiven for the surge of panic that rises upon the sight of a crimson-filled toilet bowl. But before you go racing off to the hospital, ask yourself, "What did I eat today?"

Like when you had a functioning colon, the color of what you put in your body influences the color of what comes out. The main difference now that you've gotten rid of that pesky colon altogether and are instead passing food through a j-pouch, is that any discoloration will happen much quicker. Rather than seeing the result of those beets the next day, you may see them in a matter of hours— a much shorter time than you would expect. And in the early days when both paranoia and frequent bowel movements reign supreme, hysteria is a completely understandable reaction.

Be prepared to see carnage if you eat or drink any of the following:

- red wine
- beets
- licorice
- red Jell-O®
- tomato sauce
- any food with food coloring
- iron tablets
- spinach

BULKING (YOUR STOOL, NOT YOUR MUSCLES)

When you have a j-pouch, the frequent loose stools, especially in the first year, are a nightmare. While you may find eating bran cereal is enough to slow things down, adding a bulking agent to your diet can thicken your stool, reduce the frequency with which you go, and absorb some of the digestive enzymes which damage your skin. Bulking agents are also an effective and natural alternative to antidiarrheal medications.

TYPES OF BULKING AGENTS

NATURAL PSYLLIUM FIBER
Sold commercially as Metamucil®, Konsyl®, Fiberall®, Isogel®, Fybogel®, Regulan® and Hydrocil®, psyllium (also known as ispaghula) is available as powdered drinks, capsules, bars, granules, or wafers.

STERCULIA
Known as Normacol® in granular form.

INULIN
The active fiber ingredient in FiberChoice® tablets.

CELLULOSE
Sold as UniFiber®, cellulose is an insoluble fiber powder.

METHYLCELLULOSE
A synthetic fiber usually sold as a powder or capsule under the name Citrucel®.

POLYCARBOPHIL CALCIUM
Sold as Fibercon® and Mitrolan®, and available as a pill or chewable tablet.

TIPS FOR USING BULKING AGENTS

- Start with a single dose a day and increase as needed. Do not exceed the recommended dosage.
- Take thirty minutes before eating to maximize absorption of digestive enzymes—any later than that and you'll reduce your appetite.
- Don't overdo it. If you feel constipated, are going to the bathroom much less than you normally would, or are having to strain, stop bulking until your movements loosen up.
- Take your dose without the recommended extra liquid, unless you feel you've over-bulked.
- Do not take if you suspect you have a blockage.
- Stop taking if you develop side effects including itching, severe gas, stomach or abdominal pain, nausea or vomiting.
- You may find you are particularly gassy for the first few days, but this is usually temporary.

PROBIOTICS

Probiotics are a frequent topic when you have a j-pouch, and their usefulness in helping prevent pouchitis is hotly debated. Proponents hail them as being a crucial factor in prevention, while others insist there is no evidence they make any real difference. The truth likely lies somewhere in the middle.

Because the exact cause of pouchitis isn't known, the specific role of probiotics and whether or not they help isn't clear. Like many natural treatments, probiotics seem to work very well for some people, not at all for others, and mostly, they seem to work for some people, some of the time. Clinical studies into pouchitis have yielded mixed results as to their effectiveness, yet all seem to agree that even though probiotics cannot prevent a bout of pouchitis, or stop it once it's started, they certainly do no harm. In other words, probiotics won't stop you from ever getting pouchitis, but at the worst, they may burn a hole in your wallet, and at best, they *may* help lessen the severity of your symptoms.

Probiotics can be prescribed by your doctor (VSL#3 is considered the gold standard), or you can buy both live or dormant strains from health food stores.

If you do decide to supplement your diet with probiotics, do it properly:

DO YOUR RESEARCH
Probiotics can be very expensive, and not all formulations are covered by government healthcare or insurance. And because they are not considered to be a drug, the contents of most probiotics are not regulated.

GET THE RIGHT ONE
Get a formulation that includes as many of the following as possible:

- *Bifidobacterium breve*
- *Bifidobacterium longum*
- *Bifidobacterium infantis*

- *Lactobacillus acidophilus*
- *Lactobacillus plantarum*
- *Lactobacillus paracasei*
- *Lactobacillus bulgaricus*
- *Streptococcus thermophilus*

LIVE CULTURES ARE BEST

Live cultures are more expensive and need to be kept refrigerated, but they are also thought to be the most effective.

KEEP A DIARY

Record how you feel daily for a few weeks before you begin taking probiotics, then for a few weeks after. Keeping track will make it easier for you to determine whether or not the probiotics are helping.

INFORM YOUR DOCTOR

Let your doctor know that you plan to take probiotics, and which ones you are going to take.

A SPOONFUL OF SUGAR

SURVIVING HEALTHCARE PROFESSIONALS

HEALTHCARE PROFESSIONALS AND YOUR J-POUCH

When you have a j-pouch, dealing with healthcare professionals can be frustrating. The most common issues you are likely to encounter include the following:

IGNORANCE OF YOUR CONDITION
Unless your family doctor or nurse is a specialist or has a lot of experience in gastroenterology, they will likely have only a general understanding of your condition and how to best treat it. Some general physicians may be reluctant to deal with you, and it can take days, weeks, or even months to see a specialist—you may wait a long time to get treatment. This lack of detailed knowledge on behalf of the doctor can be a nightmare if you have a bout of pouchitis that desperately needs antibiotics. Granted, most doctors are merely exercising prudence, but it can be difficult to accept this attitude when the doctor in question is refusing to prescribe you needed medications even though they can see on your chart how you have been treated in the past. There is some satisfaction when these doctors try to palm you off on to a specialist who then tells them exactly what you told them six hours ago, but that satisfaction is small.

BEING DISMISSIVE OF YOUR CONDITION

Even dealing with a specialist can be upsetting at times. They likely treat a number of patients whose conditions are more serious than yours, and you may feel that their level of concern is disproportionate to how awful you are feeling. Whether due to perspective their part (chances are, they *do* have a lot of patients who are worse off than you), or just a crappy bedside manner, don't take it personally. Try to keep your situation in perspective and remember that although they can have all the theoretical training in the world, unless they've experienced your condition for themselves, they can't truly understand it from your point of view.

RIGIDITY OF TREATMENT PLANS

You've heard that coffee enemas are a cure for pouchitis, and since it's a natural treatment, you would rather squirt liters of coffee up your butt than subject yourself to a load of chemicals. You can't understand why your doctor doesn't think this is a good idea, and obviously, they're a big meanie for not exploring this with you.

There may be a time during your illness when you want to try alternative therapies that you *know* worked for other people. (Dear, sweet Internet, you'd never lie, would you?) Many doctors will be open to you trying alternative treatments alongside your conventional ones if you can present it to them in a well thought-out pitch. Bear in mind, however, that although they are not infallible, specialists have spent a lot of time and energy learning about your condition and how to treat it, and they prescribe certain medications because, in most cases, those treatments work. If nothing else, they don't want to look incompetent, so they are unlikely to make you take anything they don't genuinely think will help . Likewise, if they tell you that all you'll get from a coffee enema is sepsis, respect them enough to listen.

TIPS FOR COPING WITH HEALTHCARE PROFESSIONALS

- Keep your expectations for care within your doctor's scope. They are not psychologists (unless they are). One professional deals with one set of issues.
- If you have chronic pouchitis, ask your doctor for a standing prescription or extra refills so that you can treat yourself if necessary.
- Have your regular doctor recommend a course of treatment in your chart, in case you become ill in their absence.
- If your doctor has the personality and empathy of a wet fart, don't take it personally. It's tough being awesome all the time.
- If you feel that you aren't being cared for properly, speak up. You may need to find another doctor.
- Be reasonable and realistic regarding the amount and type of care you expect.
- Accept that there might not be a perfect fix, and that "well" is sometimes "well enough."
- Take as much responsibility for your own care as you can.
- Express yourself in a reasonable way. Being demanding or rude will get you nowhere. Understand that, galling as it may be, your doctor holds the power, and you need them on your side.
- A perky attitude can go far in helping you to receive better care. Don't be too perky, however, or the doctor may think there's nothing wrong with you.
- If you have to cry, cry pretty.
- Your doctor is more likely to be flexible with your treatment if you are confident and capable in your self-care. Make sure you are knowledgeable, concise, and doing everything you can to keep yourself well outside of their help.
- Be willing to take advice, even if you're fairly certain it won't work for you. Your doctor or nurse will be more responsive if they feel you're trying.

- Take your medication. Yes, you may hate it or think you don't need it, but nothing will annoy a doctor more than if you refuse to follow your treatment plan and then bitch because you're not feeling well.
- That said, if you really don't agree with your doctor's plan, then don't follow it. Sometimes you do know better. Proceed with caution, however, because you may need to justify your decisions.

THE SHOW MUST GO ON

EXERCISE AND YOUR J-POUCH

EXERCISE AND YOUR J-POUCH

You may be thinking that, finally, after everything you've been through, you are no longer obligated to exercise. 'Fraid not. Coping with your j-pouch is much easier when you are as healthy as possible, and regular exercise reinforces your health in many ways:

MINIMIZES YOUR RISK OF OBESITY
A lot of extra weight can be hard on your j-pouch.

STRENGTHENS YOUR ABDOMINAL MUSCLES
Strong abdominal muscles will reduce your chances of developing a hernia.

GIVES YOU MORE ENERGY
More energy will help to combat your fatigue.

REDUCES STRESS
The endorphins produced by exercise will also help you sleep better.

AIDS DIGESTION
Exercise will help keep food moving through your system and can reduce any heartburn you may feel, especially in the first few months.

IMPROVES AND MAINTAINS YOUR BONE HEALTH
Weight-bearing exercises will help keep your bones strong.

TIPS FOR EXERCISING WITH A J-POUCH

- Although you will have to start from scratch after your surgeries, the good news is that you should eventually be able to resume an exercise regimen similar to what you had before your illness and your ostomy.
- Be cautious about exercising in the heat since you will become dehydrated quickly. Drink plenty of water or oral rehydration solution before and during exercise.
- Avoid substantial abdominal exercise for at least eight to twelve weeks after your take-down surgery—give yourself time to heal properly.
- Begin with gentler exercises such as swimming, walking, Pilates, or yoga. These types of exercise will help you strengthen your abdominal muscles while not putting too much strain on your surgery site.
- Be realistic about what you can achieve. Pushing yourself past a sensible point may set you back.
- Wear an abdominal support garment, such as a support belt or spandex, for the first few weeks of exercise. Avoid extra-tight spandex; the pressure on your abdomen may make you feel nauseous.
- Avoid contact sports for at least twelve weeks, just to be on the safe side.
- Apply a moisture-barrier cream to your butt-crack to avoid butt-chafing from butt-sweat.
- Pelvic floor exercises are an excellent way to improve continence.
- Avoid high-impact movements such as running or aerobics in the early months—you don't need any help being sore or incontinent.

- Wear a diaper or pantyliner in the first few weeks, just in case of leakage. Eating a few marshmallows about half an hour before you start exercising can also help.
- Make sure your pouch is as empty as possible before you begin.
- Take your survival kit.
- Know the location of any bathrooms along your route.

PELVIC FLOOR EXERCISES

You likely consider anal continence a desirable commodity, and pelvic floor (Kegel) exercises can go a long way in helping you achieve it. As a bonus, doing Kegel exercises before and after your surgery also tightens your urinary and vaginal (or penal) muscles, bestowing you with the ultimate trifecta of desirability.

HOW TO PERFORM THE KEGEL EXERCISE

1. Wait several weeks after your surgery before beginning or resuming the Kegels. Check with your doctor first to ensure you're good to go.
2. Locate the proper muscles by squeezing your sphincter as you do when you're desperately trying not to shart yourself. Clenching your cheeks is a bonus, not the focus.
3. At first, it may be easier to practice your Kegels while you are lying down. Lying down in bed with Netflix and a pound of chocolate makes it especially easy.
4. Tighten your pelvic floor muscles and hold for five seconds.
5. Relax for five seconds. Repeat.
6. Do four sets of five holds per day.
7. Keep breathing.
8. Work your way up to holding it for ten seconds, in sets of ten. Do this four times a day, forty clenches in all.
9. Once you become an expert at the basics, try practicing your Kegels without moving any muscles except your pelvic floor. No buttocks, thighs, abdomen, or face.
10. You can now perform your Kegels anywhere—at supper, at the movies, riding in your carriage—just remember to keep those face muscles neutral if you're in public.
11. Reap the benefit of pristine undies.

LIFE IS A HIGHWAY

TRAVEL AND SOCIAL EVENTS

TRAVEL AND YOUR J-POUCH

You may find traveling with your j-pouch easier than when you had active disease (unpredictable) or your ostomy (higher maintenance). However, preparation is still important to ensure both that your ass is covered and that you have a good time.

TIPS FOR SUCCESSFUL TRAVEL

BEFORE YOU GO

- Learn your destination country's local language for directions to the bathroom.
- Fill a prescription of antibiotics, just in case you get a bout of pouchitis while you are away.
- Obtain a prescription note to show to security if needed.
- Ensure you're aware of the bathroom situation at your destination. Especially if it's the early days of your j-pouch, you may need to go to the toilet frequently (and explosively). Many countries have Western-style toilets, some don't. Make sure you're confident to go on a squat toilet if that's what's available. Even if you feel confident, you can always practice with a bucket beforehand.
- Get decent medical insurance. Even though you are "better," your pouch could still give you problems. Be honest on your

application.

- Know where the local hospitals are.
- If available, download a bathroom locator app for the country you're visiting.

ON THE PLANE

- Book a seat on the aisle and near the toilet if you can.
- To make sure you get enough to eat on a long-haul flight, buy or bring your own snacks, especially if you have recently begun adding foods back into your diet. If you are further along in your recovery, whatever the airline is serving should be fine.
- Take a full set of your current medications on the flight with you, and put another set in your check-in luggage in case of loss.
- Bring your survival kit. If you don't want to pack your whole kit, wipes and skin cream are essential.
- Gravol® or other anti-nausea travel medications can make you sleepy and will also give you slight constipation, reducing the number of times you'll need to use the toilet.
- Bring a bulking agent to further slow things down. Marshmallows are also handy.
- Pantyliners or diapers can be useful as a security measure—you never know how quickly you'll be able to get to the bathroom, especially if there is a line. Or, go whenever there's not a line, whether you really have to go or not.
- Bring a change of bottoms, just in case.
- Buy water after you go through security so you can stay hydrated. An electrolyte powder or drink is also a good idea (just avoid bringing baggies of powder through security).
- Bring your own soft wet-wipes. Airplane toilet paper can be awful, especially if your skin is sore.

IN THE CAR

- Map out the bathrooms en route.
- Take a portable camping toilet, so you can make a dignified pit stop if necessary.
- Stay hydrated, but not too hydrated. If know you won't have many chances to stop, reduce your intake accordingly.
- Keep your kit within easy reach.
- If you recently had surgery or have pouchitis, wear a pantyliner or diaper to help accommodate any accidents.
- Don't over-tighten your seatbelt.
- Go to the bathroom whenever you have a chance, even if you don't really have to go.

ONCE YOU'RE THERE

- Have fun with what you eat—you are on holiday, after all— but not too much fun.
- Try to avoid food poisoning at all costs. Avoid buffets, and use your judgment with street vendors. Pack snacks just in case your options are limited.
- Caution foods are still caution foods when you're on holiday, and an obstruction is the last thing you want in a foreign country.
- Avoid traveler's diarrhea by being extra careful with water hygiene, including ice cubes. Traveler's diarrhea is especially bad for someone with a j-pouch.
- Keep copies of your documents on hand at all times, including a description of your condition, a list of your medications, your doctor's name and phone number, and your insurance details.
- Keep change on you at all times, just in case only pay toilets are available.
- Keep your survival kit close by.

SOCIAL EVENTS

If you're still recovering from surgery, or you're ill with pouchitis, socializing is not as straightforward as it once was. With a little foresight and planning, however, it can still be just as fun.

TIPS FOR STRESS-FREE SOCIALIZING WITH A J-POUCH

- Get your outfit ready the day before, plus a back-up. This way you will not be stressing at the last minute.
- Bring your survival kit. If your kit is large, pare it down to the bare essentials or carry travel sizes.
- Do a bathroom reconnaissance when you arrive. Know where the bathrooms are so you don't have to run around frantically looking for them when you do actually need to go.
- If you're at a restaurant, don't make a big production about what you can and can't eat. If you can't eat the mushrooms, fine. You don't have to order them. Nor do you have to explain to everyone WHY you can't order them. Just choose something else.
- If you're having a meal at someone's house, let your host know ahead of time what you can't eat. Otherwise, you risk making them feel awkward when you can't eat what they're serving.
- Eat slow, small, and what you know. Don't take risks just because it's a special occasion.
- Don't get wasted. Being blind drunk can increase your risk of accidents.
- Don't talk about your illness all night. The whole point of going out is that everyone enjoys themselves. Don't ruin it by boring everyone to death. If somebody asks, fine. But keep it brief and clean.
- Always have an exit strategy. If the people you're with know about your condition, you don't need to make excuses—just

tell them you don't feel well and leave. If they're unaware of your situation, decide in advance how much (or little) you want to tell them, or just say you have a headache.

- If you have an accident while you're out, deal with it and try not to let it ruin your night. Having an accident in public can be daunting, but if you're prepared, you can sort it out quickly. Don't let the fear of accidents at any stage of your illness keep you from going out. If you're having a particularly bad case of pouchitis, take preemptive action by wearing a diaper.

- If you're obligated to attend a social event while you have pouchitis, standing around, walking, or dancing may not be activities you feel capable of doing. Just sit at your table and let people come to you. You'll look much cooler that way, anyway.

SOMEBODY THAT I USED TO KNOW

THE EMOTIONAL IMPACT OF A J-POUCH

EMOTIONAL IMPACT OF A J-POUCH AND HOW TO COPE

Many people view their j-pouch as the conclusion of their illness, the final step in a long and painful journey. You no longer suffer an embarrassing yet invisible illness. You no longer have an external pouch that is a constant reminder of your condition. You can now perform even the most basic human function normally. Your life becomes your own again.

Right? …Hello?

Unfortunately, this (completely forgivable) optimism can make the emotional impact of living with a j-pouch more overwhelming than it should be. Having a j-pouch is a wonderful, terrible blend of hope and disappointment, victory and defeat. The anticipation of your brilliant new life, the realization of those moments that actually live up to it, and the times when, after all you've been through, you get kicked in the teeth yet again. It's not a voyage for the faint-hearted.

Some people can absorb the hysteria and take it in their stride. Other people struggle more at this time than any other time in their illness.

PRE-SURGERY CONCERNS

You may have mixed feelings about your anastomosis or take-down surgery including:

FEAR

- You might be worried about whether or not the operation will be a success—usually, you get only one shot at an internal pouch.
- You might be afraid of leaving behind the relative security of your stoma.

ANXIETY

- You might be concerned about coping with the long recovery period, especially if you don't have a strong support network.
- You may worry about the negative implications that the surgery might have for your future, such as the effect on your fertility.

EXCITEMENT

- You may be so excited about finally "getting your life back to normal," that you give exactly zero f**ks about the surgery.

POST-SURGERY CONCERNS

After your surgery, you may experience any or all of the following:

CHANGES IN BODY IMAGE AND SELF-ESTEEM
You may:
- Be distressed at your new abdominal scars. J-pouch scars never go away, and many don't get lighter with time.

- Become more body confident if you were self-conscious about your stoma.
- Find you are more confident and happy with your body now than before you developed your illness.
- Even love your new scars, rejoicing in them as the well-deserved battle-trophies they are.

FRUSTRATION

You may be frustrated at:

- The slowness of your recovery. Remember: months to years.
- Experiencing complications such as pouchitis, setting your recovery back just as you were beginning to feel better.
- Not feeling as well as you thought you would. Some people think that a j-pouch will make you "normal" again. It doesn't.

REGRET

You may regret:

- Having the surgery. You may feel that you were happier and healthier with your stoma.
- Putting yourself through surgery because you underestimated your recovery progress. You may resent the time that healing will take and the uncertainty that you will ever be as well as when you had your stoma.

ANXIETY ABOUT YOUR QUALITY OF LIFE

You may feel anxious that:

- You're not, and won't ever be, as active as you were before the surgery.
- You may struggle to conceive.
- You will become sick again and need to have further surgery, or that you will face a lifetime of complications, medications, and illness.

- Your illness and resulting treatment is only the beginning; you're constantly waiting for the other shoe to drop.

FEAR

You may be afraid that:

- Your pouch will be unsuccessful, and you will need a permanent stoma.
- You will never really be well, or as well as you hoped or expected to be.

DEPRESSION

You may find all of the frustration, regret, anxiety, and fear becomes overwhelming. If you have suffered depression previously, you may constantly be afraid it will return and wonder how you will cope. Signs that you may be depressed include:

- Being unwilling or unable to care for yourself properly.
- Finding it difficult to speak to anyone about what you are feeling or to seek help.
- Being unable to cope with things you would have had no trouble with before.
- Over or underreacting to situations.
- Withdrawing from your relationships and support network.
- Feeling suicidal.

COPING WITH THE EMOTIONAL IMPACT OF YOUR J-POUCH: METHODS, PROS, AND CONS

Before getting a j-pouch, you had to deal with both illness and having an ostomy; you've got a lot of experience with coping. The coping techniques for living with your j-pouch are likely similar to those you've already been using, so you should have an idea of which strategies will work for you:

THE VETERAN
(You survived, now you're moving on.)

Pros:

- Pushing yourself forward can, at this late stage, actually go a long way in helping you to recover. You have endured the spectrum of whatever your condition had to offer, and although you still have to deal with the implications of it for the rest of your life, you've technically won the war.

Cons:

- You may find yourself becoming overwhelmed at unexpected times, over relatively trivial things.
- People may assume that you are "better," and may not realize that you are still dealing with a different quality of living and will be for the rest of your life.
- People may not understand the enormity of what you went through and may underestimate both the emotional and physical toll it has taken on you.

TALKING TO FRIENDS AND FAMILY
(It's been a magical journey.)

Pros:

- Speaking to the people who have known you before and during the process of your illness can help you work through what you're feeling. You may find it interesting and valuable to hear what other people think of the progress you've made.
- Letting people know your current needs and limitations is helpful to both you and them. Since your pouch is now internal, your condition has become invisible again, and as a result, some people's expectations for you can be unrealistic.
- People tend to be much more comfortable with the idea of the internal pouch and that you can "go to the bathroom normally" now. As a result, they are often more open to discussing what has happened to you. They see you as

recovered, so your illness may no longer be a sensitive topic or an issue that will continue to be as prevalent in your lives.

Cons:

- Because you no longer have external signs of your condition, some friends and family may be ready to move on from talking about it.
- You may have already spoken at such great length about your illness that people are no longer interested.
- You may not like to hear what people have to say, especially if their view of your progress differs from yours.

RESEARCH YOUR J-POUCH

(Since you may as well know *EVERYTHING*.)

Pros:

- Knowing a lot about your pouch can make you feel more prepared, and this can help you to cope better and may help your recovery go smoother.
- Knowledge can increase your confidence even when your recovery feels slow.
- Understanding your condition can put your recovery in perspective. You may be doing better than you thought, or you may realize that you are struggling needlessly when there are solutions available.

Cons:

- Too much knowledge can lead to anxiety about complications that may never happen. There is more information available regarding negative outcomes than positive ones since they take longer to discuss than simply saying "I/they/we/the patient feels great."
- Some of the statistics, such as those for reduced fertility, can be unnecessarily discouraging.

J-POUCH FORUMS
(You should be a full-blown netzien by now.)

Pros:

- Like when you had your illness and your stoma, speaking to other people in your situation can be very helpful.
- Forums are great for practical advice on life with your j-pouch, especially when you are experiencing complications.
- There is a low level of commitment—you can drop in or out as you wish.
- You may find that you can begin to help other people who are struggling.

Cons:

- As with your original condition and your stoma, if you are looking for general information on living with a j-pouch, the forums can present a disproportionate amount of negative experiences. While it is useful for you to be aware of these experiences, they can be disheartening to your recovery, especially when you are in a difficult place.
- Forums can sometimes lead you down a rabbit hole of self-pity.
- Forums can have a culture of one-upmanship over who has it worse, making you feel as though your legitimate concerns are insignificant.

PERSONAL BLOGS
(A j-poucher's account of their experience, from diagnosis to present-day.)

Pros:

- You get a comprehensive view of what life can be like with j-pouch—including the ups as well as the downs.
- Personal blogs can be a great source of inspiration.

Cons:

- Each blog represents only a single person's experience. You may want specific information that isn't covered by that particular blog.

J-POUCH SUPPORT GROUPS
(More like the Goonies than Fight Club.)

Pros:

- You are a member of a very exclusive club now, and it can be fun to get together with the other members and NOT talk about your condition. You may find that unless one of your members is having a particular issue, you rarely discuss your condition itself and instead spend your time talking about your plans for the future.
- Some groups arrange for different therapists or other professionals to come and give talks, for example, sex therapists or cocktail mixologists.

Cons:

- Having a j-pouch is uncommon, so unless you live in a very large city, you'll probably be the only person in your town with one. That said, why not have a meeting with yourself, take yourself out for a nice dinner?
- If one person in the group is really struggling with their recovery, it can become a delicate situation. Issues such as fertility can cause tension that members may struggle to cope with. Likewise, some pouchers want to talk about the future—they're through with having their condition play a large role in their lives and want to move on—while some need more time to reflect in order to recover.
- Sometimes members who are doing well can be somewhat impatient with those who are having issues.

PROFESSIONAL HELP
(The night is dark and full of terrors.)

Pros:

- A therapist can give you an extra level of support, especially if you've spent much of your time until now surviving rather than coping.
- Some people find that anti-depressant or anti-anxiety medication can boost their recovery; often it is something they only need short-term. Others may find that they need it longer.
- Talking to someone you don't personally know can help you explore feelings that you may feel uncomfortable discussing with your family, especially if your loved ones think you are coping well, or if they can't understand why you aren't coping better than you are.
- Professional therapists have experience in dealing with anxiety issues such as post-traumatic stress.

Cons:

- You may feel that your experience is too unique to be helped by someone who has not gone through a similar event.
- Some people feel that there is a stigma attached to seeing a therapist.
- You may feel uncomfortable or unjustified seeking help because you are "cured."

RELATIONSHIPS AND YOUR J-POUCH

Throughout your experience with illness, the dynamics of your relationships have likely changed, and having a j-pouch is no different. Even though the impact of your pouch will likely be less profound than when you were diagnosed or when you had an ostomy, your j-pouch can affect your relationships in both negative and positive ways.

NEGATIVE EFFECTS ON YOUR RELATIONSHIPS

PEOPLE THINK YOUR J-POUCH IS A "CURE"

And technically, it is. For *active large bowel disease*. In reality, you are trading a greater evil for a lesser one. You will continue to have issues with your health, whether autoimmune or from the pouch itself. This can be difficult for people to understand, especially since there are few outward signs of your condition. You may also find that people become dismissive of everything you have gone through to get to this point, and this can be extremely frustrating.

PEOPLE OVERESTIMATE THE RESTRICTIONS OF YOUR J-POUCH

Conversely, having your insides reconstructed is very mysterious to people, and some will continue to treat you as though you're an invalid when you're not. Often, their greatest concern is that your pouch will become damaged and you will have to go back to the ostomy bag. The more they know about your condition, the more overbearing they may become. (*"According to my list here, you shouldn't have nuts. No cake for you!"*) People tend to see your condition as black and white, not realizing that the experience and adaptation of having a j-pouch is different for everyone.

KIDS NO LONGER GIVE A CRAP, UNLESS YOU SHOW THEM YOUR SCARS

Your scary/cool reign has come to an unceremonious end. Scars, although imbued with street cred in their own right, don't have quite as much impact as an ostomy bag. If you tell them you got the scar wrestling a cougar, however, they'll still think you're a boss.

YOUR PARTNER MAY COME CRAWLING BACK
If you became estranged from your spouse (or from any of your friends, for that matter) because your illness was inconvenient for them, now is the time they may come slithering back. Think long and hard if reconciliation is what you need or even want. What would happen to the relationship if your j-pouch had to be reversed?

POSITIVE EFFECTS ON YOUR RELATIONSHIPS

THE KID GLOVES COME OFF
Even though some people may continue to be overbearing, especially in the short-term, you may find that most people relax a bit and aren't as focused on your condition. Even though people have your best interests at heart when they're coddling you, you may find that it's wonderful to be 'normal' (well, your version of normal, anyway) again.

YOUR MARRIAGE MAY REGAIN SOME EQUILIBRIUM
It's not that your marriage will get better per se, but if your spouse treated you like a delicate flower because of your ostomy, now is the time you'll get your groove back. Likewise, if your spouse was uncomfortable (rightly or wrongly) with your ostomy, now will be the time they get their shit back together.

COPING WITH CHANGES IN YOUR RELATIONSHIPS

BE VERY CLEAR ABOUT YOUR NEEDS AND LIMITATIONS
Let people know (diplomatically) what you can and can't do, and what you need and don't need from them. Everyone can relax once they

know where they stand.

ANSWER PEOPLE'S QUESTIONS
Many people find the idea of a j-pouch fascinating. Don't be surprised or offended by people's questions about your j-pouch, no matter how awkward they are. Unless the person is *trying* to make you feel awkward, then be as offended as you like.

ACCEPT THAT THE PEOPLE WHO COULD NOT DEAL WITH YOUR ILLNESS OR YOUR OSTOMY MAY WANT TO BE FRIENDS/LOVERS AGAIN
Whether you want them back is up to you, but don't compromise yourself for someone who isn't worth it.

POST-TRAUMATIC STRESS AND YOUR J-POUCH

Only recently has post-traumatic stress been associated with illness. The term usually conjures up images of events considered far more extreme, such as combat and sexual assault. Even those people who suffer from significant illness hesitate to place their experience in a similar context; however, post-traumatic stress is becoming recognized as a very real effect of both acute and chronic illness.

CAUSE OF POST-TRAUMATIC STRESS IN J-POUCHERS

THE THREAT OF DEATH OR SERIOUS INJURY
Post-traumatic stress is characterized by anxiety caused by exposure to trauma such as the threat of death or serious injury. In that context, having your colon removed and facing the prospect either of living permanently with an external bag or having an unpredictable organ created by cutting up a perfectly healthy one can surely be considered traumatic?

YOU CAN'T PREPARE FOR IT
Another cause of PTS in the ill is the trauma caused by a profound sense of helplessness and compounded by a lack of preparedness. In his article *How PTSD Became a Problem Far Beyond the Battlefield* (Vanity Fair, May 7, 2015), Sebastian Junger notes that highly-trained soldiers were found to have lower rates of PTS than their less-prepared counterparts. There is no training to prepare you to spend your life fighting debilitating illness.

YOUR ENTIRE LIFE CHANGES, *AGAIN*
Missing the war when it was finally over was another source of PTS addressed by Junger. It wasn't that soldiers missed the combat itself, but rather the "closeness and cooperation that danger and loss often engender." The close bonds you may have forged with others over your disease suddenly are no longer relevant. You no longer receive

the same standard of medical and familial attention, and the focus shifts away from you and the illness which has defined and influenced every aspect of your life for so long. You are no longer 'sick,' but nor are you "cured." It's easy to feel as though you have been abandoned in an uncertain No Man's Land of living one day at a time.

SYMPTOMS OF POST-TRAUMATIC STRESS

- anxiety and depression
- insomnia and nightmares
- agitation, jumpiness, and difficulty concentrating
- feeling extremely vulnerable
- guilt, shame, and self-blame
- hypervigilance about your health
- emotional numbness and disinterest
- avoidance of certain persons, places, or things that you associate with your illness
- making uncharacteristic decisions
- flashbacks or physical reactions such as sweating, dizziness, and increased heart rate when thinking of your surgery or defining moments in your illness
- inappropriate emotional responses such as irritability or anger that are out of context for the situation
- substance abuse as a coping strategy
- physical pain that doesn't respond to medication

OBSTACLES TO RECOVERY AND DIAGNOSIS

Although accepted in the medical community, a diagnosis of post-traumatic stress can be difficult to both accept and recover from. Obstacles can include:

GUILT AND SHAME
Some j-pouchers resist a diagnosis of PTS because of feelings of guilt and shame. You may feel that the seriousness of your condition in relation to others, such as those suffering from cancer, or those events

traditionally associated to PTS, does not warrant such a grave reaction. You may feel like a fraud or failure, as though you are asking for more attention and sympathy than you deserve—no matter how bad your condition may be, it isn't terminal. You will survive, and you may feel a certain level of guilt if you feel anything but happy and grateful.

THERE ARE SOME POSITIVE ASPECTS TO THE EXPERIENCE

About studies done on the recovery of soldiers and rape victims, Junger notes that "combat is generally less traumatic than rape but harder to recover from." This is in part, he believes, due to rape being an acute, solely horrific and traumatizing event, whereas the experience of combat is a prolonged situation interwoven with a strong sense of community and camaraderie, an experience that can be as sweet as it is bitter. This narrative can be applied to illness—pain, fear, and long recovery periods interlaced with the happiness, love, and hope of daily life.

SOCIETY BELIEVES YOU ARE LESS

Perhaps the largest obstacle to recovery from post-traumatic stress is the understanding and reaction of society. In the soldier's case, stress can result from leaving a close-knit community with common understanding, goals, and support, and reentering a culture that is comparatively individualist. In the case of ostomates and j-pouchers, trauma can be intensified by our culture's devaluation of those who are chronically ill, especially when it comes to an invisible illness.

Contrary to public chatter, our culture is very impatient with recovery. There is a stigma towards being chronically ill or disabled, a shamefulness associated with dependence. As noted by S. Kelley Harrell, the sick are expected to "miraculously recover or die. That's the extent of our cultural bandwidth for chronic illness." We value the appearance of health over the individual, and as a result, there is a marked lack of understanding and empathy towards those who are chronically ill which can result in their alienation from not only society, but from friends, families, and partners.

TIPS FOR COPING WITH POST-TRAUMATIC STRESS

The following tips are based on personal experiences only; they are not a substitute for professional advice.

Many people find that having therapy for their post-traumatic stress is crucial to their recovery. If you think you are being affected by PTS, discuss your options with your doctor.

But whether you are having therapy or not, there are lots of small ways you can cope with PTS on a daily basis:

MAKE CONNECTIONS

If you have a good support network, talk to your family and your friends. They have been there through your illness, and they may have some insight into the source of your PTS and how to help you. If talking to your family or friends isn't helpful, you may find that dedicated support groups and forums are. If you don't want to talk, you don't have to, but don't isolate yourself—do something with someone, it doesn't matter what.

EXERCISE YOUR BODY

Many people recovering from PTS have noted how helpful physical exercise actually is. Not only can it help you feel good and make you sleep better, but it can also help you to cope with your physical reactions to the stress. And yes, dancing around your living room counts, but getting out of the house is better, even if it's only going down the street to buy a Cronut. And the best? Getting out into some good old-fashioned nature.

EXERCISE YOUR MIND

When you're doing something, live in the moment of whatever you're doing; pay attention to what's going on outside of yourself. This doesn't mean ignoring what's going on inside your head, just take time off from focusing on it. Find a new hobby that you really enjoy—it won't stop your stress from surfacing, but you may eventually find that it begins to translate into something more positive and productive.

DON'T AVOID IT

One of the best ways to deal with PTS is to be prepared. Figure out what your triggers are. It may be tempting to avoid them, but facing them in a controlled way, at your choosing, can help you overcome them. Practicing breathing exercises can help you to control your response when you do trigger it. Keep a journal to track your progress. Reward yourself with another Cronut.

IT'S OKAY TO BE SAD AND ALONE

Take the time to be alone and quiet. Constantly surrounding yourself with noise will make it impossible to face what you're going through. Put on a sad song or movie, and ugly cry. Don't forget something happy for after.

USE A CRUTCH

While you are coping, it's okay to use small tricks to help you get by. Develop a mantra to repeat to yourself, or carry a talisman—anything that stimulates a sensation that you find pleasant, such as perfume, a tactile object, or a photograph. When everything starts to go tits-up, say it, smell it, lick it, whatever.

MAKE YOURSELF VISIBLE

Invite people to share your experience with you. Write a personal blog (or even a book), contribute to forums, give talks to increase awareness about your condition, run a marathon. You will be *seen*.

TALK DIRTY TO ME

SEX, PREGNANCY, AND YOUR J-POUCH

SEX AND YOUR J-POUCH

J-pouchers seem to have mixed reactions towards sexuality. Some find themselves reinvigorated, some carry on as normal, and some despair at the thought of probing of any kind. Most, however, feel more comfortable with their bodies once they no longer have the external bag.

PHYSICAL CHANGES AND ISSUES

Physical changes associated with an ileo-anal anastomosis can be temporary or permanent, and can include any of the following:

VAGINAL DRYNESS
Dryness can be due to nerve damage during surgery.

ERECTILE DYSFUNCTION
Like vaginal dryness, erectile dysfunction is also caused by nerve damage during the surgery.

DECREASED SENSATION IN YOUR CLITORIS
Also due to local nerve damage.

PAIN
Penetrative sex may be painful the first few times due to scar tissue and dryness—many j-pouchers find this to be temporary.

DECREASED LIBIDO
Due to all the medication, surgery, and your changing psychology, sex may be the last thing on your mind.

PRESSURE ON YOUR POUCH
Significant pressure on your pouch can be very uncomfortable.

RECOMMENDED BAN ON ANAL SEX
Your small intestine is much less elastic than your colon, and because your pouch is usually attached directly to your rectum, penetration can result in damage to your anastomosis, and in extreme cases, pouch rupture. Some j-pouchers do continue to engage in anal sex successfully, but whether or not it is advisable for you personally needs to be discussed with your surgeon.

MINOR ANAL LEAKAGE
Leakage can be caused by pressure on your pouch.

EMOTIONAL CHANGES AND ISSUES

You may:

- feel self-conscious about your surgical scars
- feel pressured to begin having sex before you are emotionally and physically ready
- be worried about being rejected
- fear any associated pain
- just not feel sexy
- worry that your partner no longer views you in a sexual way because they have been your caretaker at times
- worry about embarrassing leakage

TIPS FOR SEX WITH A J-POUCH

- Wait at least six weeks before attempting penetration.
- Expect initial pain, and don't be alarmed if the discomfort persists for several months.
- Keep in mind that your partner's view of your sexuality in regards to your scarring and physical condition usually correlate with your feelings about it—if you're having a good time, so will they.
- Wait until you are ready, and be honest with yourself and your partner about when that is. Don't feel guilty if you're not ready.
- If your doctor advises you against anal sex, DO NOT HAVE ANAL SEX. Seriously, don't do it.
- Do whatever you did before your surgery to make yourself feel sexy.
- Engage in acts of coitus that don't involve penetration. Google it if you need to.
- Use lube. Lots and lots of lube.
- Deeply penetrative sexual positions may be uncomfortable for lady-pouchers.
- Experiment with props and toys.
- Use protection. Even though your fertility may be reduced, you can still get pregnant.
- Masturbate, with or without your partner. Masturbation can help you get used to your new body, and make you feel more confident about eventually having sex.
- Foreplay, foreplay, foreplay.
- Accept that the first time may be a bit awkward for both you and your partner.
- Start slow and small—save the sex swing for the second go.
- Don't push it (literally). Know when to stop. Cuddle. Try again later.

PREGNANCY AND YOUR J-POUCH

Anastomosis surgery is a major operation, and it can have a lasting impact on your ability to conceive. Scar tissue formation is the main culprit for reduced fertility in j-pouchers, and currently, there is no standard treatment. As fertility is thought to be reduced in some cases by as much as 50%, some ostomates delay their anastomosis surgery until they have had children. Those who have had the surgery may need to consider fertility treatment or adoption, but many do end up conceiving naturally even when told by their surgeon that their chances are slim.

While getting pregnant can be an issue for some women, the good news is most who do have normal, healthy pregnancies. And while a Caesarean section is performed in most j-poucher deliveries, a surprising number of women manage to have a vaginal birth.

The odds turned out to be in your favor, and you're pregnant. Now what?

WHAT TO EXPECT DURING PREGNANCY

- The positional pain you may experience with your pouch (if you feel intense pressure or pain when you lay on one side or the other), can change or disappear.
- You'll find that you go to the bathroom more frequently as your pouch and your baby fight for real estate. This may last only until the second and third trimesters, or it may continue throughout your pregnancy.
- Due to internal scarring, your baby may sit further on one side of your body than the other.
- Your scars *will* stretch, don't worry.
- You may experience pouchitis during your pregnancy. Although antibiotics like ciprofloxacin pose a slight risk to your baby, the complications due an uncontrolled infection pose a greater one. Discuss your concerns with your doctor, and follow their advice. Don't stress about it.

- If you have ongoing problems with your immune system, you may be put on antivirals to prevent infections such as shingles. Antivirals usually pose no risk to your baby.
- Your progress may be monitored by your doctor more frequently than if you did not have a pouch.
- Whether you are considered high-risk or not will depend on your past and present health. Your doctor will consider your medical history to determine if you are at risk of developing conditions such as pre-eclampsia.

TIPS FOR COPING DURING PREGNANCY

- If possible, find an OBGYN who has dealt with j-pouch pregnancies. Their experience enables them to offer you better advice and will help give you more peace of mind.
- Begin using Bio Oil®, or a similar product on your scars and belly the minute you find out you're pregnant. The oil will help facilitate belly expansion and prevent stretch-marks.
- Rejoice in a lack of hemorrhoids. Whether due to the lack of constipation and straining, or the webbing of scar tissue holding your baby aloft, lots of j-pouchers don't seem to get hemorrhoids. Yay us!
- Eat little and often to keep your nutrition up, especially if you have a lot of nausea and morning sickness.
- Take extra care of your perianal skin to avoid the risk of infection.
- Drink meal replacement drinks if you can't eat. If you are struggling to keep anything down, you may have to have intravenous nutritional support.
- If you're vomiting a lot, you'll become dehydrated quickly. Stay hydrated by drinking small amounts, often. If you are unable to keep liquids down, you may need to have intravenous fluids.
- Avoid caution foods that place you at a higher risk for an obstruction. It's only for a few months!

WHAT TO EXPECT WHEN GIVING BIRTH

- It is possible for some women to give birth vaginally after their j-pouch surgery, but you may be encouraged to have a C-section to maintain the integrity of both your pouch and your sphincter muscles (a tear could result in permanent incontinence). Your surgeon will evaluate your particular case and make recommendations.

- If you do have a Caesarean, your surgeon may choose to make the incision along your previous anastomosis scar.

TIPS FOR COPING WHEN GIVING BIRTH

- Don't insist on a risky vaginal delivery against your doctor's recommendations just because you feel it is more "natural." You have an internal pouch; the "natural" ship has sailed, and you are not on board.

WHAT TO EXPECT AFTER BIRTH

- You may find it takes several days for your pouch function to return to normal.
- J-pouchers have the same ability to breastfeed as non-pouchers.
- Chances are good that the positional pain you had before you became pregnant will return.
- You may get a bout of pouchitis while you are breastfeeding. Taking antibiotics while breastfeeding is not ideal, but timing feeds or expressing can minimize any risk to your baby. Unfortunately, antibiotics also have a tendency to reduce milk production; multiple bouts of pouchitis can eventually stop it altogether.

TIPS FOR COPING AFTER BIRTH

- While breastfeeding, avoid holding your baby in a position that puts pressure on your pouch. Putting a pillow between your baby and your abdomen will reduce any pressure.

ALL FUR COAT AND NO KNICKERS

J-POUCH FASHION DOS AND DON'TS

Reaching the j-pouch stage is exciting for a lot of people in terms of what they can now wear. You no longer have to plan your outfit around your ostomy, and the heady sense of freedom can be intoxicating. And as you know, intoxication can lead to bad decisions. Just because you can now wear whatever you want does not mean you can dress yourself with reckless abandon. Follow these basic guidelines until the giddiness subsides:

J-POUCH FASHION DOS

GO RETRO
Wear what you wore before the nightmare of illness began.

IF IT AIN'T BROKE . . .
If you genuinely liked what you wore during your ostomy days, continue to enjoy.

SUN HATS
To help reduce your chances of dehydration. Not necessary in winter,

of course.

SENSIBLE HEELS AND/OR STURDY SHOES
Until you get your pouch under control, you may occasionally have to run to the toilet.

STRETCH DENIM AND LEGGINGS
Especially if you like to wear fitted clothes. The stretchier, the better—you want to avoid putting too much pressure on your abdomen, especially for the first six months.

MATERNITY PANTS AND ELASTIC WAISTS
Very comfortable for the first few months after take-down. And during pouchitis. And for the rest of your life.

SWEATPANTS/LOUNGE PANTS
Soft, comfortable. There is a fine line between sleek and slovenly, and you can no longer use your illness as an excuse—unless you are actually ill, then wear whatever you want. Choose sweatpants that look as good as they feel. Think more Karlie Kloss on her day off, rather than couch-potato debutante.

BIKINI OR A ONE-PIECE
Think of your scars as a badge of honor, but if you want to avoid nosy questions or you're not comfortable showing them off, don't.

BE DARING
Try stuff you wouldn't have worn before. Abdominal scars really keep that belly sucked in, so take advantage.

TAILORED DRESSES
Anything that flares at the waist will avoid putting pressure on your tender abdomen.

DIAPERS
If you're having some leakage, such as after surgery or during a bad

case of pouchitis, don't let incontinence ruin your fun.

COTTON UNDERWEAR

You'll be making frequent trips to the bathroom, and cotton undies will help keep everything cool and dry and will absorb any excess butt-cream.

J-POUCH FASHION DON'TS

PLAYSUITS, PANTSUITS, OR ONESIES

Wait until you are in good control of your pouch. You may have to get your pants down quickly, and you also risk wiping the toilet floor with your collar.

POLYESTER PANTIES

Polyester + frequent bathroom trips + sore skin + creams = dankness + chafing + sad face.

A THONG OR A G-STRING

The *rubbing*.

FRUMPY CLOTHES

Celebrate.

WHITE BOTTOMS

At least until you are confident in your continence.

BLOOD ON THE TRACKS

J-POUCHES AND THE SHIT PEOPLE SAY

IT MUST BE SO EXCITING TO BE NORMAL AGAIN!
Well, I was "normal" before, during, and after my illness…so not that exciting.

YOU MUST BE GLAD TO NO LONGER HAVE ANY HEALTH PROBLEMS!
I've had intensive drug therapy. I've had multiple surgeries. I don't have a colon. My insides are literally stapled together. I still have the same immune system, and too much chocolate could still make me fat. Believe me, I've still got problems.

SO, DO YOU, LIKE, LITERALLY HAVE A, LIKE, BAG INSIDE YOU?
Yes, it's beautiful and pink, and I managed to get it for only a colon. Only, I can't show it off, and the only thing I can keep inside it is shit.

WHERE DOES THE POO COME OUT?
The usual place. Unlike yours, which seems to be coming out of your mouth.

HOW DO YOU STOP FROM POOPING YOURSELF?
I think about seeing you naked—that tends to tighten my sphincter right up.

CAN YOU FART? WHAT HAPPENS?
Yes, I can. It smells. And sometimes I follow through with a puff of glitter.

WHAT ARE YOUR POOS LIKE?

They're smart, funny, and love long walks on the beach.

YOU MUST BE SO HAPPY TO HAVE GOTTEN RID OF THAT AWFUL POUCH!

That awful pouch saved my life. And I could eat as many hot wings as I liked.

"YOU SHOULD JUST GET A HYSTERECTOMY" (ON LEARNING ABOUT YOUR REDUCED FERTILITY).

I will. If you promise to get a glossectomy.

WILL YOUR COLON GROW BACK?

Um…no. Nor would I want it to. Bowel disease, remember?

LOADED AND ALONE

SOCIAL MEDIA

SOCIAL MEDIA DOS AND DON'TS

Thanks to social media, you can now tell people how you're feeling the minute you feel it, but just because you can, doesn't mean you should. Posting about your illness when you have a chronic condition like a j-pouch can be tricky, especially if you have a tendency to post mainly negative comments. Occasionally telling everyone how awful you feel can be comforting as a way to both vent and get some well-deserved love thrown back your way, but constant status reports on just how hard you have it does both yourself and friends a disservice. Social media was not created for the sole purpose of providing you with a captive audience for a blow-by-blow account of the trials of your life.

Consider how you view posts on social media. Do you have a friend whose feed consists in large part of complaining about how crappy their life is? Even if their bitching is perfectly justified, after the first few posts and your sympathetic responses, chances are you've begun to dread seeing their name appear on your feed. You may feel resentful at the constant and obvious expectation for you to respond to what seems less like a sharing of feelings and more like an invitation to a self-indulgent pity-party. Since nothing you say seems to make a difference anyway, the whole exercise becomes tiresome, and you struggle to sympathize. Be honest. If you're not already ignoring that person's posts, you're probably considering it. If you don't feel this way, then you're either a saint or lying. And who could blame you? You have your own stuff to worry about.

Whether this reaction to another person's hardships is right or wrong is not the point; it's simply how the majority of people feel. While people are happy to extend kindness and compassion to someone they like or love, they also have an understandable desire to carry their own burdens. I'm not saying you shouldn't discuss your illness on social media—you should— but talk about it in a way that is inclusive rather than alienating, and you'll find that people are more than happy to give you the support you need.

DOS

BE POSITIVE
Although it can be difficult at times, try to post comments about your illness only if they are positive. Positive posts can include personal milestones you've reached, good news you've received, or goals you've achieved in spite of your illness.

BE EDUCATIONAL
Bring awareness to your illness as a whole (rather than just your personal experience of it) by posting relevant articles about topics such as new breakthroughs in treatments. People who are genuinely curious will have a look, and those who aren't can bypass them.

BE FUNNY
Humor is often the best way to let people know how you are feeling without seeming as though you want pity. People enjoy laughing, and having a j-pouch is a goldmine for universally-enjoyed potty humor. That said, keep it clever and classy—otherwise, people just think you're crude.

BE HONEST
At the end of the day, be honest with yourself. You're posting about your illness because you want attention and sympathy. That is not a bad thing; you deserve it. But do it sparingly and in a way in which

people feel they can be supportive without being obligated to carry you.

BE PART OF A GROUP
There are social media groups for people with j-pouches. If you need to vent, vent to people who can properly empathize. You may not be special, but you'll be understood.

BE REALISTIC
Don't post with the sole intention of seeing how many of your friends respond then measuring your worth against these responses or lack thereof. Social media is used by people to socialize with minimal effort on their part. Understand it as such.

DON'TS

BE SELF-PITYING
Nothing scatters people to the wind like self-pity. Self-deprecation is fine, but self-pity makes people very uncomfortable. You'll get supportive comments back from some people, but many will eventually steer clear of you. Fair? Maybe not, but it's reality.

BE ANGRY
Like self-pity, anger about your condition also makes people very uncomfortable. It's no one's fault that you're ill, not even your own. The universe doesn't give a shit, so there's no point raving about it.

BE SELF-ABSORBED
Even if you're posting positive comments about your illness, do so judiciously. People get bored of seeing that crap constantly infiltrating their timelines. You're ill. We get it!

POST SELF-INDULGENT HOSPITAL SELFIES
Thumbs up after a successful surgery? Good. Pouty face in a hospital bed that screams "I need even MORE attention than 24-hour medical care can provide"? Bad.

TRY TO BAIT SYMPATHY

Read your post aloud before you send it. It can be painfully obvious that you're fishing for attention when you think you're being easy-breezy.

TAKE IT PERSONALLY

People have their own lives to live and are usually more concerned with that than how many bowel movements you've had today. It's not that they don't care, it's... Well, it's that they don't care. It's not personal; it's cat videos.

SISTER MORPHINE

A GUIDE TO BEING IN THE HOSPITAL

HOSPITAL SURVIVAL KIT

YOUR OWN PAJAMAS
Having your own PJs makes a difference physically and psychologically. It's far more pleasant to be lying there in something soft and beautiful that you've picked, rather than an over-starched burlap bag that a hundred people have worn. If morphine makes you adventurous, definitely opt for pajama pants to guarantee your ass is covered.

WIPES
Although hospitals do have toilet paper, it ain't the good stuff. Plus, you can use the wipes for your hands, your face, etc. if you won't be getting out of bed for a while.

YOUR OWN COFFEE CUP
Make yourself at home.

PEN AND PAPER
Just think about how many classics have been written while the authors were off their tits in a drug-fueled haze. See this as your opportunity.

COMPUTER
Load it up with movies, TV, games, whatever. Try to make everything

available offline, because hospital Internet is expensive. If you can then get your eyes to focus, you're golden. If you really want to be online, but don't want to pay, bring mobile WiFi.

BOOKS, MAGAZINES ETC
Magazines are especially good since there is usually a roaring trade of swapsies. Don't bring anything too intellectual, however; due to the morphine, chances are you won't remember anything you've read.

SLIPPERS
Most hospitals are pretty clean. But still. Slippers can be especially useful in a surgical or GI ward—there is sometimes blood and other accidents. Get some with good grips.

MIRROR, TWEEZERS, MANICURE SET
Being in the hospital may be the only time you get to pamper yourself, so take advantage.

HAIRBRUSH AND HAIR ACCESSORIES
It's purely psychological. Plus, single doctors and nurses.

SOAP, SHAMPOO, AND YOUR OWN TOWEL
You can get this stuff from the hospital, but your own is so much better.

BATHROBE AND SHOWER SHOES
Trying to get dressed again in a wet shower room is the *worst*.

MENSTRUAL PADS
Yes, the hospital does supply menstrual pads, but unless you enjoy wedging a comically large brick of cotton between your legs, bring your own.

YOUR TEDDY
Just make sure you wash it when you get home.

PHOTOS

Photos of your family serve as a memento of what you have to look forward to when you get out. This reminder can help make your hospital stay more bearable, especially if you can't stand some of them.

A HOBBY OF SOME KIND

You never know how long you may be in the hospital. I became a cross-stitch adept due to the amount of time I spent inside.

MOISTURIZER

For some reason, hospitals are really damn dry.

MONEY

For bribes and the mobile snack cart that delivers bedside.

RULES OF HOSPITAL ETIQUETTE

YOU ARE NOT STAYING AT A HOTEL
Before you complain about the food, the 'service,' or even the lighting, stop and think about where you are. If you're well enough to complain about everything, you're well enough to go home.

NURSES ARE NOT SERVANTS
I understand that the uniforms are confusing. I know that you're scared, and you're sick, and you're in pain. So am I. And yet, I don't feel that it gives me the right to be an asshole. If you can haul yourself out of bed and down the hall to have a cigarette, don't soil the bed because it is "the nurse's job" to wipe your ass. Have some respect.

SHUT UP
I'm avoiding eye contact with you for a reason. The curtain is drawn around my bed for a reason. I'm pretending I'm dead *for a reason*. That reason is that I don't want to talk to you. If you just wanted to say "Hi," great. "Hello!" But you don't. You want to tell me your life story, and you want to hear mine, and I am sorry, but I am just not interested. My sympathy well has run dry. I am tired, and in pain, and I just want to watch *Game of Thrones*.

HAVING SEX IS NOT APPROPRIATE
Ever.

TAKE YOUR MEDICATION
Nobody is going to give you a gold star for being tough and not taking your pain meds, but I *will* punch you in the teeth when you start whining because you're what? In pain? Also, NOBODY LIKES HEPARIN. But you'll like a thrombosis even less, I promise.

DON'T BE MELODRAMATIC
People may die right in front of you. It's sad and scary and awful. But don't make it about you and your feelings, *especially* when their loved

ones are there.

WASH
If you can't make it to the shower on your own, get the nurses to help you. I understand that we're all a bit stinky on the GI and surgery wards, but there's a limit. I inadvertently laid in my own filth for two days while temporarily paralyzed after my first surgery, and neither the nurses nor I noticed the smell because the woman in the bed next to mine had refused to wash for *days*.

YOU'RE NOT THE ONLY PATIENT ON THE WARD
You may be in a ward with patients whose illnesses are more serious than yours. (Hard to imagine, I know.) Make your needs clear, but not every five minutes. The nurses will get to you as soon as they can, if for no better reason than to shut you the hell up.

DO NOT MAKE YOURSELF UP AND SPEND YOUR TIME TAKING POUTY SELFIES
This makes you look like an asshole at any time, but *especially* at this time.

A "THANK-YOU" BASKET FOR THE NURSES AFTER YOUR STAY WOULDN'T GO AMISS
And not a crappy fruit basket either.

HOW TO ENJOY YOUR STAY

TRY TO THINK OF IT AS A HOLIDAY
You are encouraged to take free narcotics. You get to choose your meals from a menu and have them delivered to your bedside. Your linen is changed daily. You can sleep whenever you want. It may not be the best holiday you've ever had, but you did pay for it in blood, tears, and taxes, right? You might as well enjoy it.

UNDERSTAND THE SYSTEM
Stock up on breakfast items. Breakfast tends to be the best meal of the day—after that, things can get weird. Fill the drawer in your little nightstand with as many peanut butter packets and bananas as you can, even if you hate bananas.

BEHOLD THE MYSTERIOUS TAPESTRY OF HUMAN LIFE
Some of the strangest shit you'll ever experience will be in the hospital. Roll with it. If a lady thinks you're her husband and tries to get into bed with you, choose to think it's because her husband has fabulous, perky breasts and not because you have a steroid beard. Don't take it personally if she later tries to stab you with a butter knife.

IT'S HOBBY TIME!
You finally have some free time to enjoy your hobbies. Knit, make lists, or finish Skyrim.

BINGE WATCH/READ
Catch up on every book, TV show, or movie you always wanted to enjoy.

WRITE LETTERS
Having to look your mortality in the face may make you re-evaluate your life. Write letters to people and tell them the things that you have always wanted to tell them. Especially if you want to tell them you

think they're an asshole. They need to know, and you may not get another chance.

YOU HAVE NO CHORES
Except eat, maybe walk a few steps, and keep yourself clean. Easy.

YOU HAVE AN ADJUSTABLE BED
Up, down, slanty, flat—lots of people would kill to have one of these at home.

YOU'LL GET SYMPATHY GIFTS
Everyone who visits you in the hospital feels they should bring gifts— unless they're horrible. Yes, you will probably get a lot of grapes, but you'll get some good stuff too, I promise.

PRACTICE PASSIVE-AGGRESSION
If you're not fond of the person who is visiting, you can always pretend to fall asleep. Stare into space for a few seconds, mumble, "Thank you so much for coming to see me . . . " and down you go.

CLOSE YOUR CURTAIN
Enjoy the peace and quiet.

BOND WITH YOUR FAMILY MEMBERS
Get your significant other to become your shower boy/girl. They'll get to feel helpful, and you'll get to be scrubbed down by someone who has already seen you naked. Try not to look too sexy (see Rules of Hospital Etiquette).

MAKE FRIENDS, OR NOT
You can meet some very nice, interesting people in the hospital, especially if you share a condition. At the same time, don't feel that you have to be social with anyone. Just focus on getting yourself ready for the rest of your life.

COWGIRLS DON'T CRY

TOUGH LOVE RULES FOR SURVIVING YOUR J-POUCH

IT'S OKAY TO FEEL SORRY FOR YOURSELF, BUT DON'T BE OBNOXIOUS ABOUT IT
Self-pity is destructive and even worse, boring.

SYMPATHY IS FICKLE
Don't milk it.

BE PATIENT
In the beginning, your frequent bowel movements will feel like bowel disease all over again, but your pouch will expand, and you will eventually make fewer trips to the bathroom. Just don't expect it to happen straight away.

USE A BULKING AGENT
Fiber is not just for old people. You may find that a couple of doses a day make all the difference to your life as a j-poucher by helping you go to the bathroom less frequently, more firmly, and with a lot less burn.

DIAPERS HAVE COME A LONG WAY SINCE YOU FIRST WORE THEM
Use them. Get over it.

GIVE IT TIME, BUT DON'T WASTE THAT TIME ON REGRET

If you regret having your anastomosis, remember that it's reversible. You usually get only one shot at having the pouch, however, so give yourself time to consider.

BE REALISTIC

Have realistic expectations for your recovery and quality of life. A j-pouch is not a perfect fix. Even without complications, it's a long, hard road.

KEEP A DIARY OR A BLOG

You'll be able to see how far you've come.

CONSIDER YOUR FUTURE

Use your recovery time to evaluate your life in terms of what you can do and what you want to do, not what you can't do or what you've lost.

DON'T GET COCKY

Just when you think your recovery is going well, it won't. One day at a time.

BE PROACTIVE

If you're struggling, take a closer look at things you might not think are important, such as your diet. Not being proactive about your own care is a choice—you have no one to blame but yourself if you don't change the things you are able to.

BE SELFISH WHEN YOU *NEED* TO BE

This does not mean all the time.

USE A COMBINATION OF COPING STRATEGIES

Do what works for you, not what other people say you should be doing.

RESPECT THE BURN
Food will come out at least the same level of spicy as when it went in. Not concerned? Rub a bit on your eyeball first and see how that goes.

SCARS ARE AWESOME
You only get them if you survive something. Don't be precious about it.

YOU ARE MUCH MORE BOTHERED ABOUT THE WAY YOUR BODY LOOKS/SOUNDS/SMELLS THAN ANYONE ELSE
Really.

REMEMBER:
If you're not feeling even a tiny bit of illness, pain, nausea, sadness, anger, fatigue, irritation, itchiness...

IT'S BECAUSE YOU'RE DEAD.

ACKNOWLEDGEMENTS

Love to my family and friends, as always. Thank you for your compassion and sympathy swag. I especially like soap and chocolate. We all thought this stage was going to be the easiest—thank you for your support when it wasn't.

Extra thanks to Peter Foong and Adam Smith, whose insight and feedback was invaluable in building this book, and to Mia Darien, for her excellent work.

To my surgeon, thank you for doing a far better job than you expected to.

APPENDIX

SURVIVAL KIT CHECKLISTS

*For printable checklists, go to screamingmeemie.com

J-POUCH SURVIVAL KIT CHECKLIST

- ☐ wipes
- ☐ Vaseline®
- ☐ mentholated lotion
- ☐ antidiarrheals
- ☐ painkillers
- ☐ change of underwear
- ☐ change
- ☐ scent spray
- ☐ pantyliners
- ☐ antibacterial hand wipes/gel
- ☐ moisturizer
- ☐ bulking agents
- ☐ a list including your condition, medications, and doctor's details

HOSPITAL SURVIVAL KIT CHECKLIST

- ☐ pajamas
- ☐ wipes
- ☐ coffee cup
- ☐ pen and paper
- ☐ computer
- ☐ books and magazines
- ☐ slippers
- ☐ mirror, tweezers and manicure set
- ☐ hairbrush and accessories
- ☐ soap
- ☐ shampoo
- ☐ towel
- ☐ bathrobe
- ☐ shower shoes
- ☐ menstrual pads
- ☐ teddy
- ☐ photos
- ☐ hobby supplies
- ☐ moisturizer
- ☐ money

GLOSSARY

anastomosis: The juncture where your pouch is attached to your anus.

cuffitis: Ulcerative colitis that just won't die.

ileoanal pouch anastomosis (IPAA): What you've got. Also called an ileoanal pouch, ileal-anal pull-through, or even a restorative proctocolectomy. The connection of an internal pouch made from your small intestine to your anus.

j-pouch, s-pouch, w-pouch: What us cool kids call our IPAA. Named for the shape of your pouch.

j-poucher: You, and anyone else with a j-pouch.

obstruction: A blockage of your small intestine or pouch, most commonly due to adhesions or food particles.

perianal skin: The skin around your anus. Potentially a source of great despair.

pouchitis: An infection in your pouch. Almost like ulcerative colitis.

stricture: A narrowing of your pouch that causes an obstruction.

take-down: The surgery that closes up your loop ostomy and basically plumbs you in.

INDEX

Made in the USA
Las Vegas, NV
18 January 2022